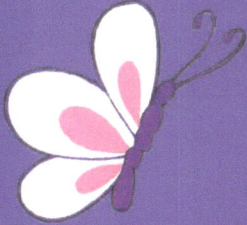

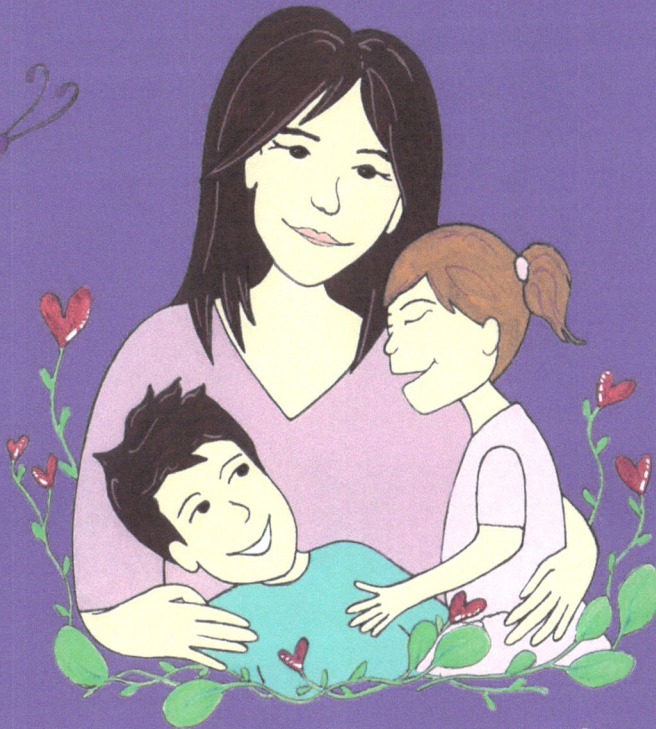

Soft Hugs for Mommy

Learning to live with Fibromyalgia

Words by Mandy D. Farmer

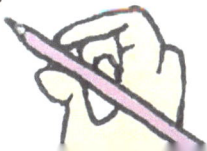

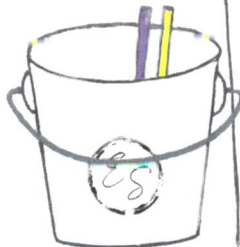

Illustrations by Melissa G. Pickens

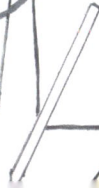

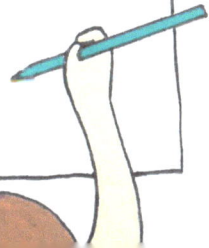

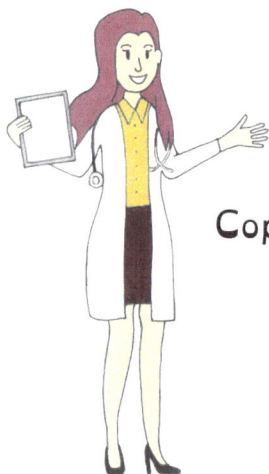

Soft Hugs for Mommy
Learning to Live with Fibromyalgia
Mandy Dawson Farmer

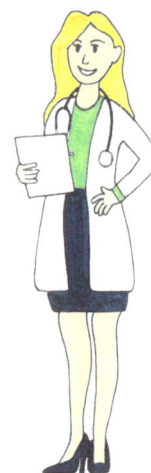

Cover Design: Melissa G Pickens
Illustrations: Melissa G Pickens

This book was prepared for publication by Evelyn Sherwood Publishing, LLC. No part of this book may be reproduced without express permission from the author Mandy Dawson Farmer.

If seeking permission to reproduce any portion of this book, please contact the author at author@mandyfarmer.com

Library of Congress Control Number: 2024921382

ISBN: 979-8-9891666-9-5

evelynsherwoodpublishing.com

Dedication

To my doctors at Mayo Clinic – Jacksonville who helped diagnose and treat my chronic pain for the first eleven years, without whom I would be in a world of hurt.

Thank you, Dr. Benjamin Wang & Dr. Mark Hurdle

To my Lord and Savior, Jesus Christ.

"Not to us, O Lord, but to You goes all the glory, for Your unfailing love and faithfulness."
Psalm 115:1 NLT

And to my husband, Michael Farmer, who has cared for me selflessly all these years. He has taken our wedding vows to the nth degree, taking on laundry, meals, and many other household chores, not to mention hours of driving and sitting with me through doctor appointments and surgeries. He has been the most committed and compassionate man a gal could dream of. Without him, I could not have made it this far.

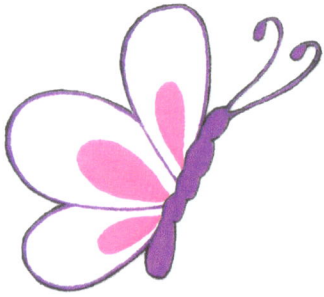

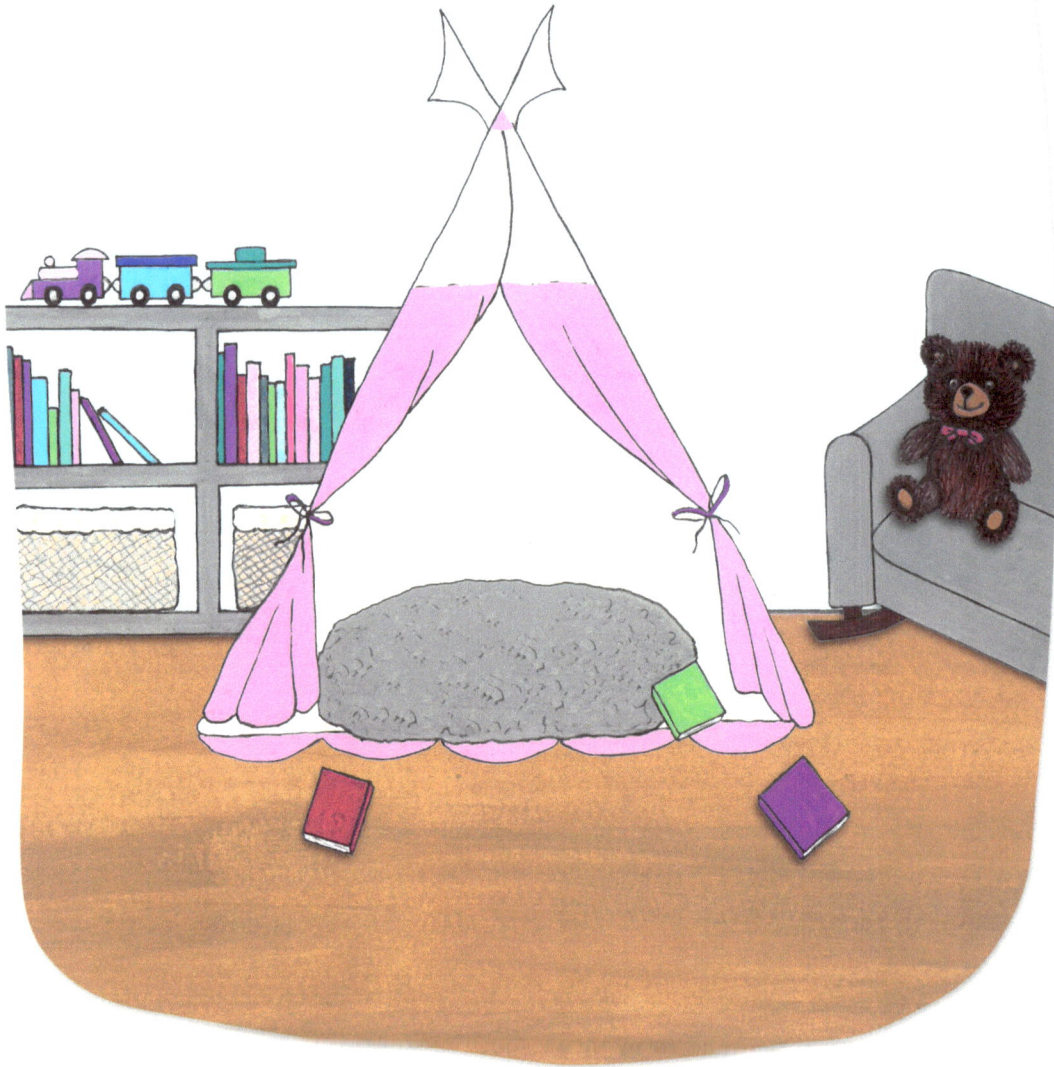

What is Fibromyalgia (Fibro for short)?

Fibromyalgia makes a person feel achy and sore all over their body. It hurts even if someone taps on their arm. Sometimes people with fibromyalgia also feel tired, but they have a hard time sleeping.

Although Fibro can make someone feel bad, it's important to know that it is not contagious. You cannot catch it.

Sometimes when a person has Fibromyalgia, they need to rest a lot. It's really important for them to have love and help from their family and friends so that they can feel better and manage their symptoms.

Purple represents Fibromyalgia! When you see a purple ribbon, it is a reminder of people with Fibro. Look for hidden purple ribbons in this book. How many can you find?

Check your answers in the back!

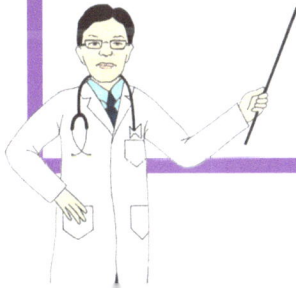

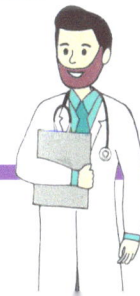

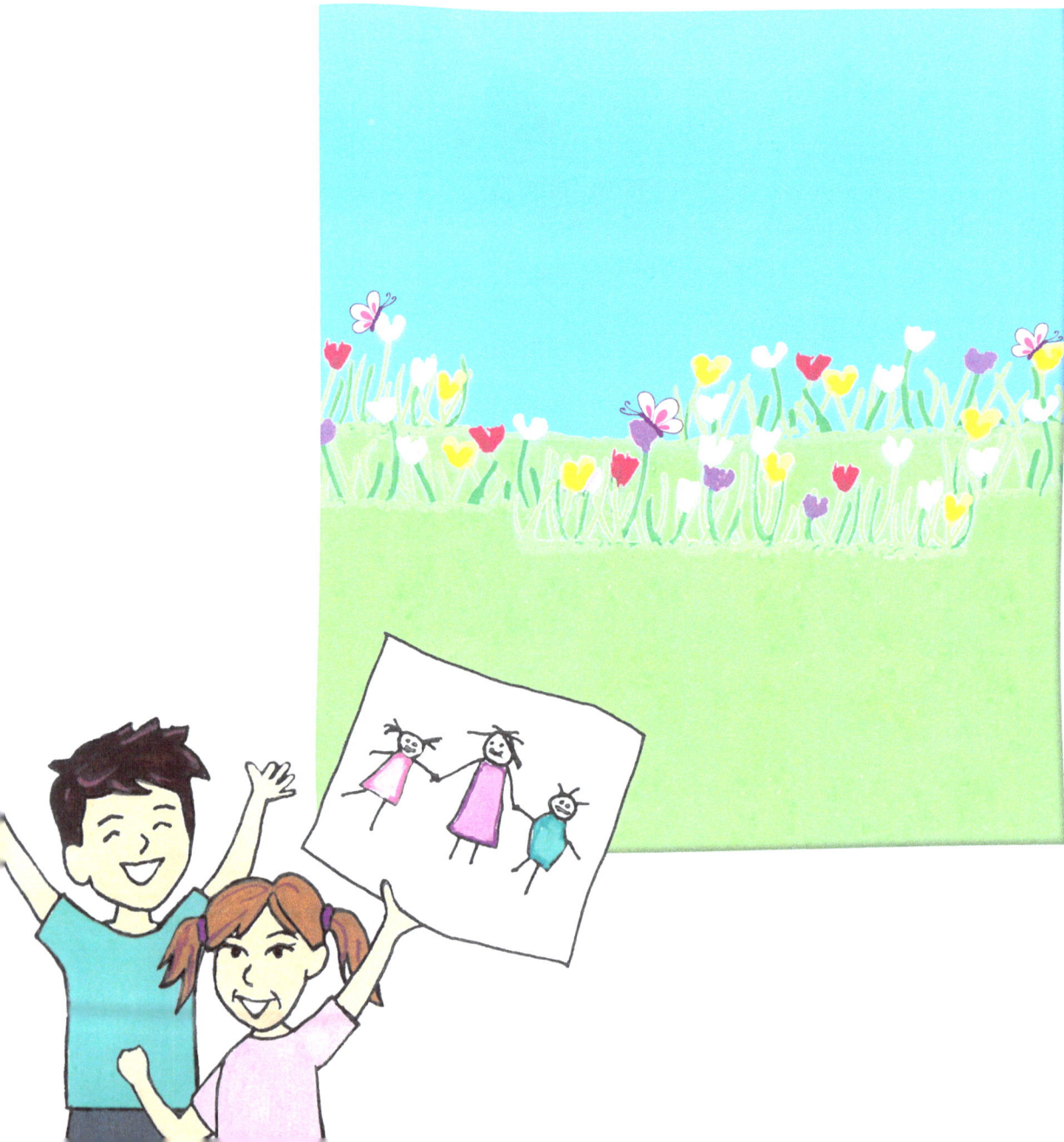

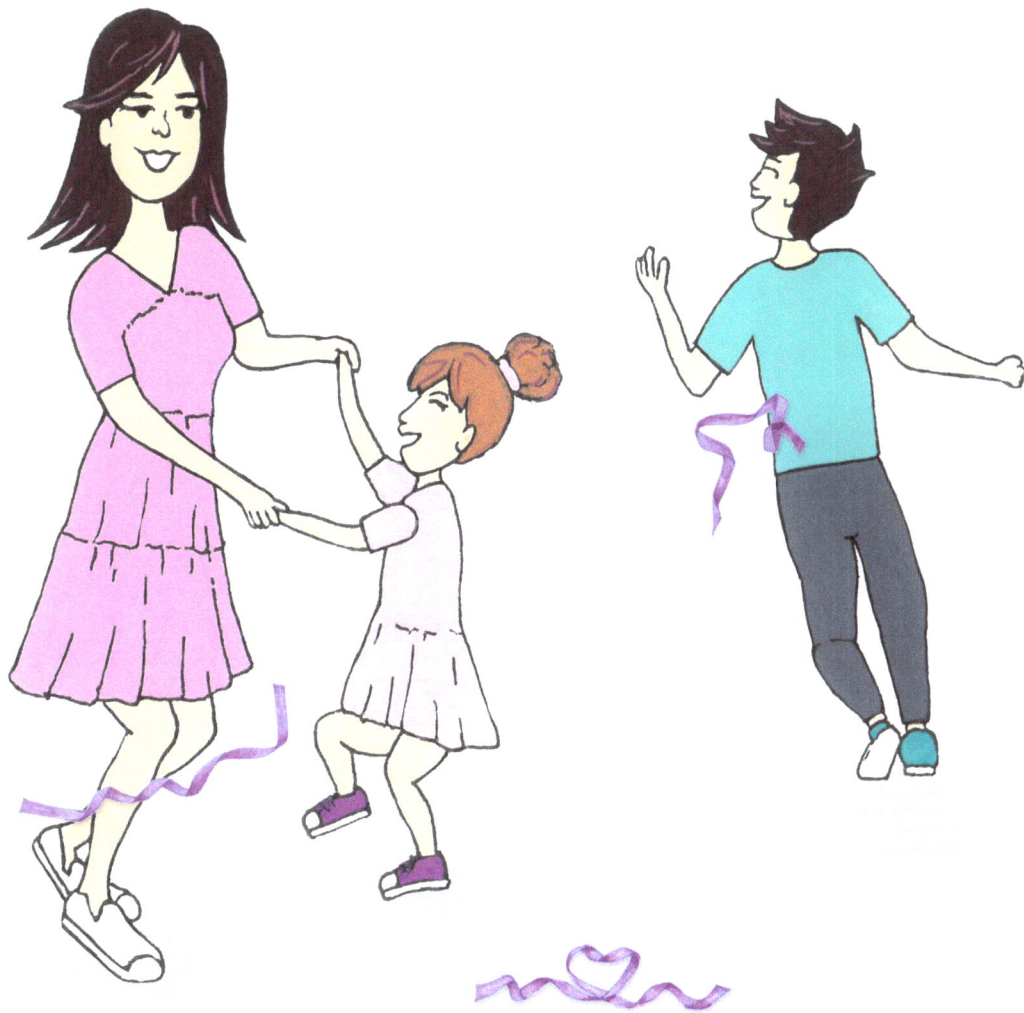

My mommy is the best mommy ever.

She loves my brother and me this much.

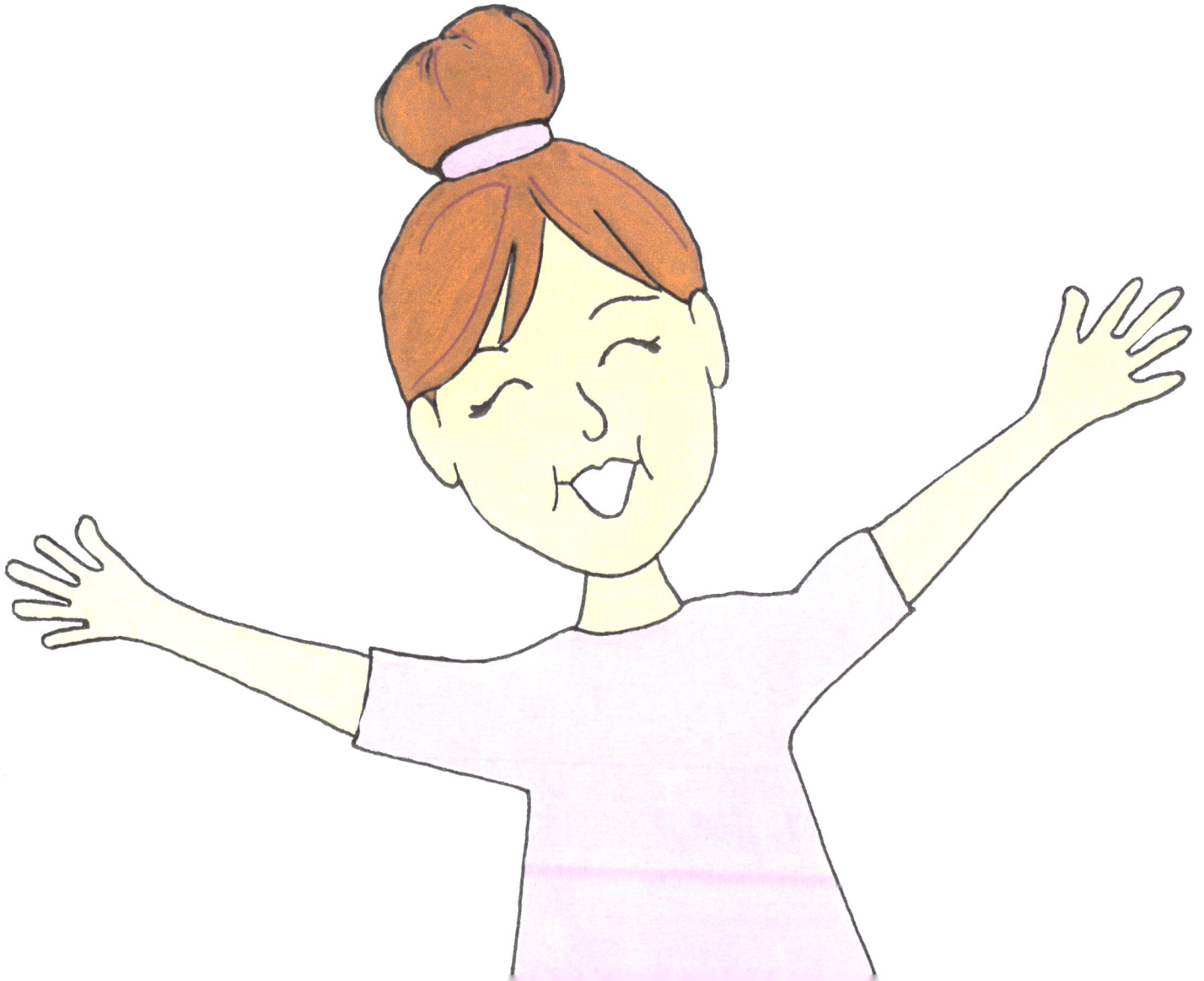

She used to give us big bear hugs.

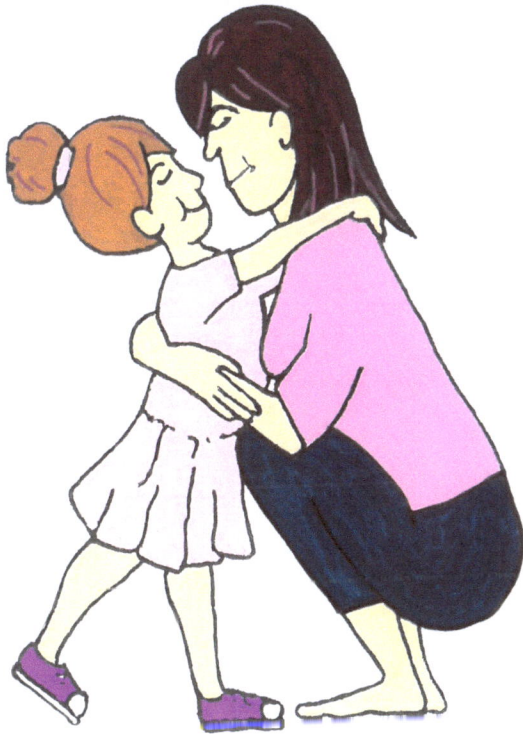

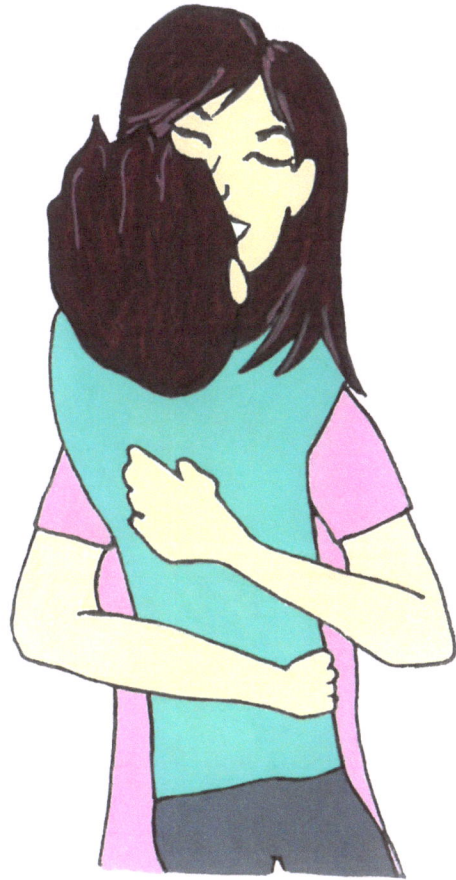

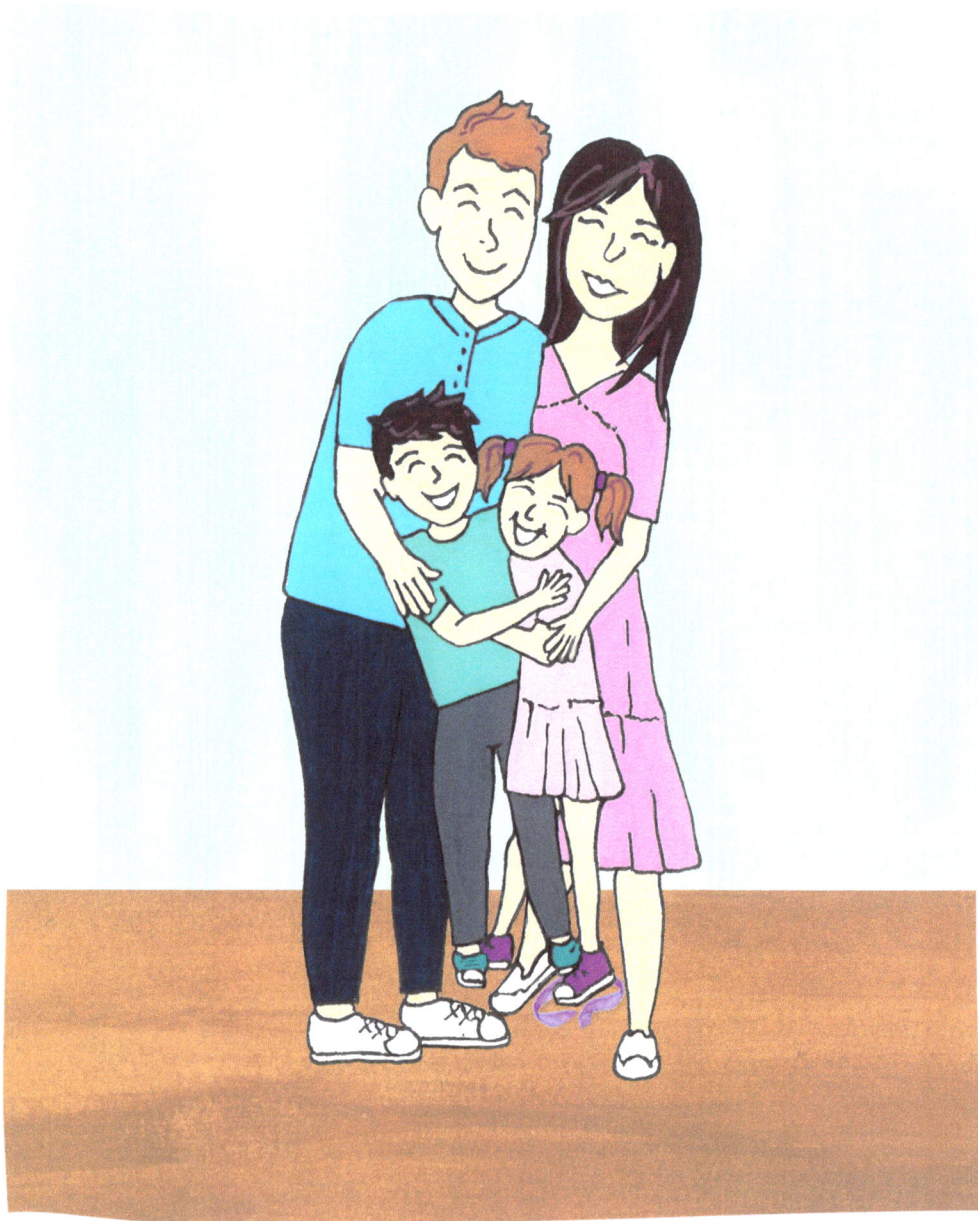

When Daddy came home, we got sandwich hugs.

But not so much now - Mommy's arms hurt.

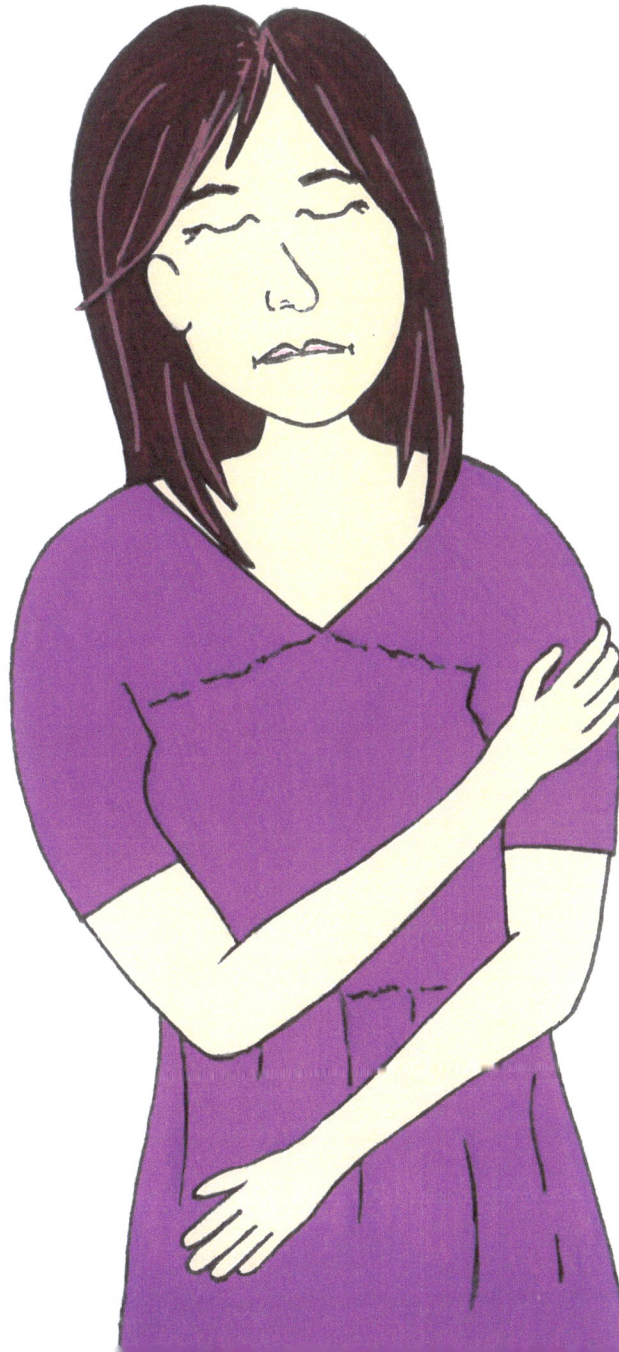

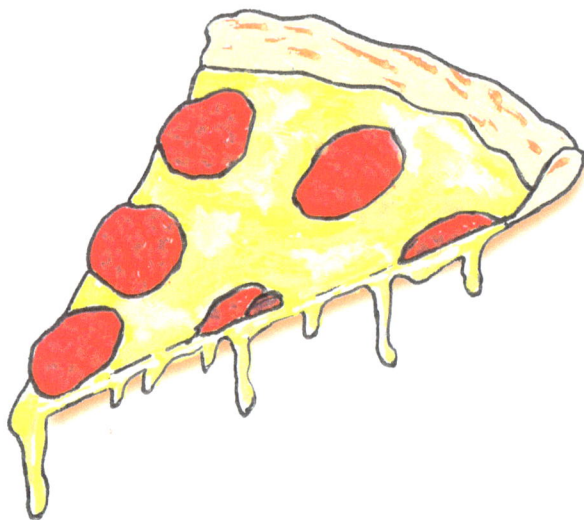

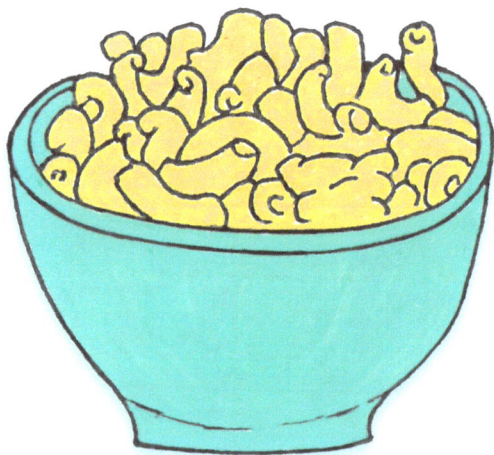

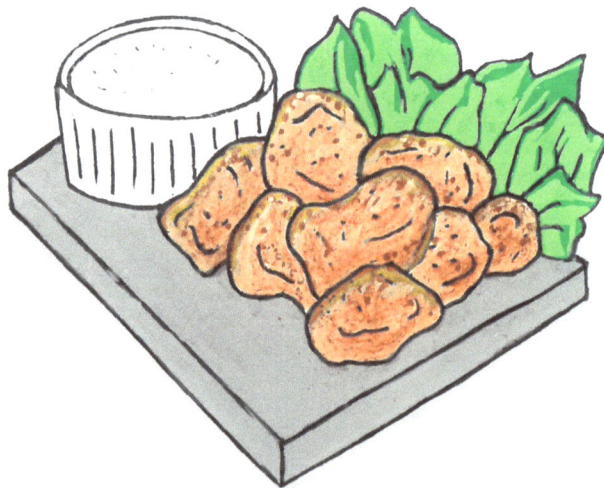

She fixed us great meals.

But now her back hurts, and she stays in bed.

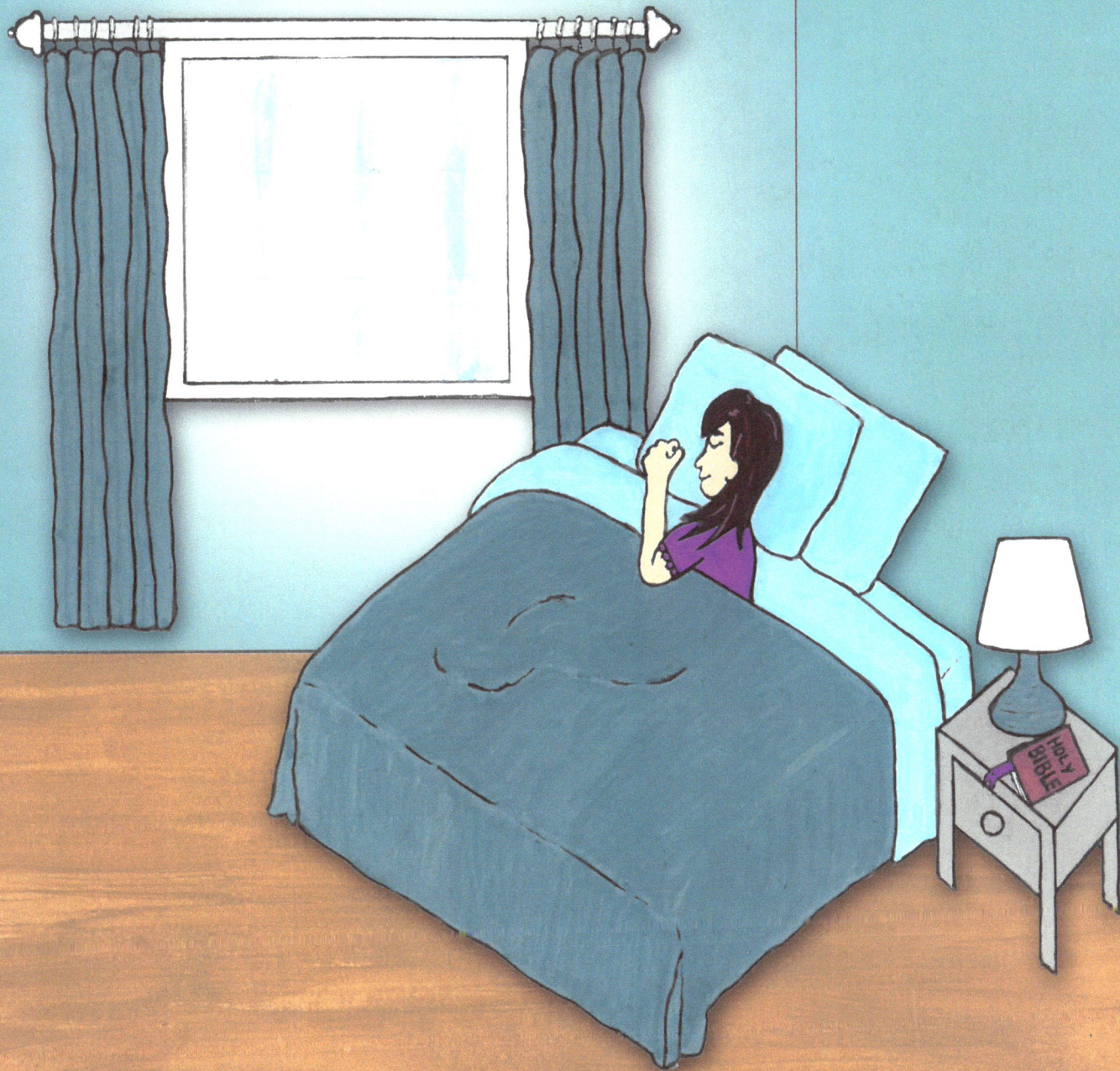

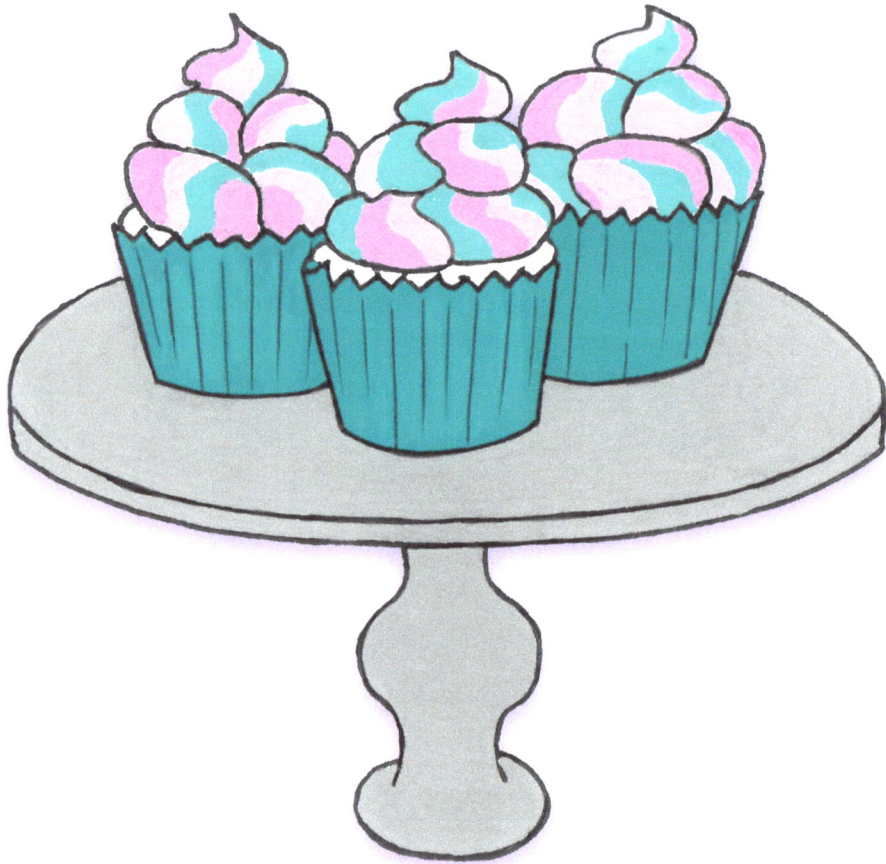

She also made us yummy treats!

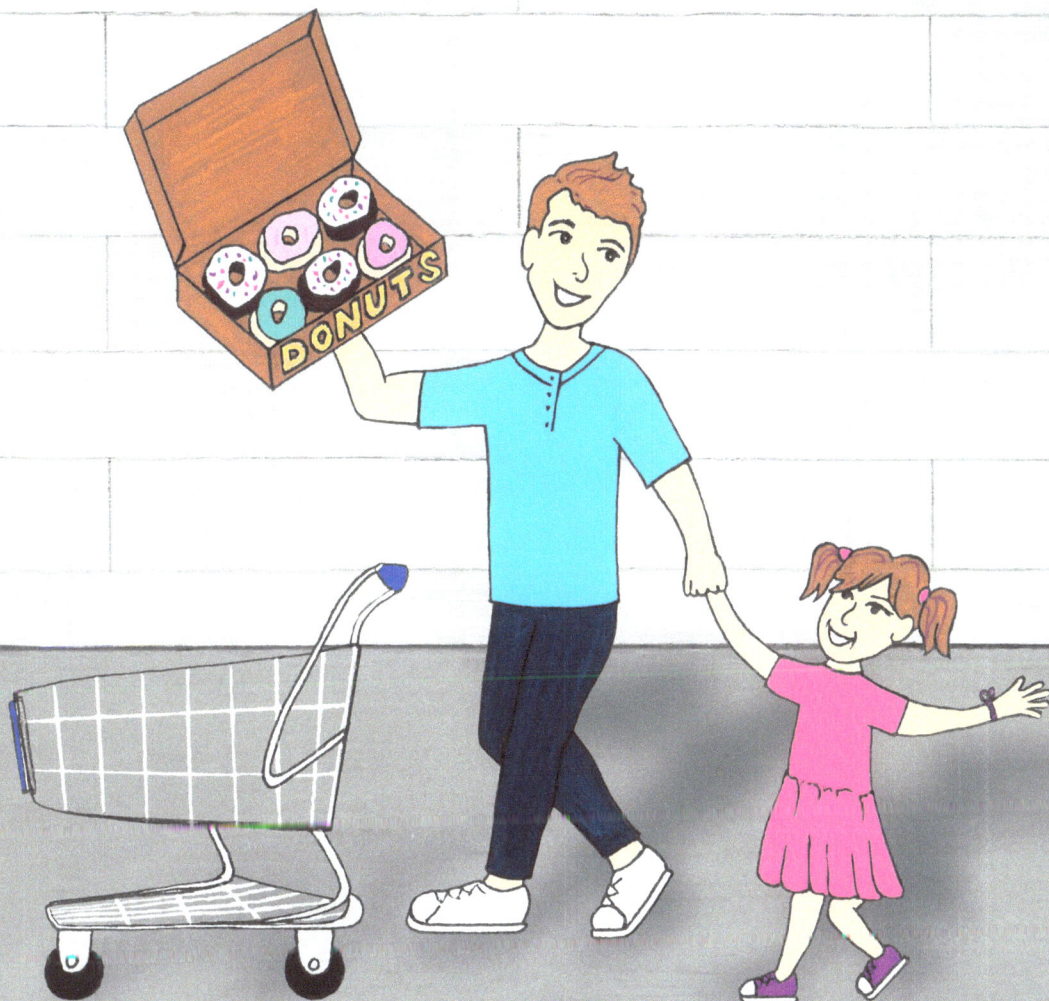

BAKERY

Now, Daddy brings treats from the store.

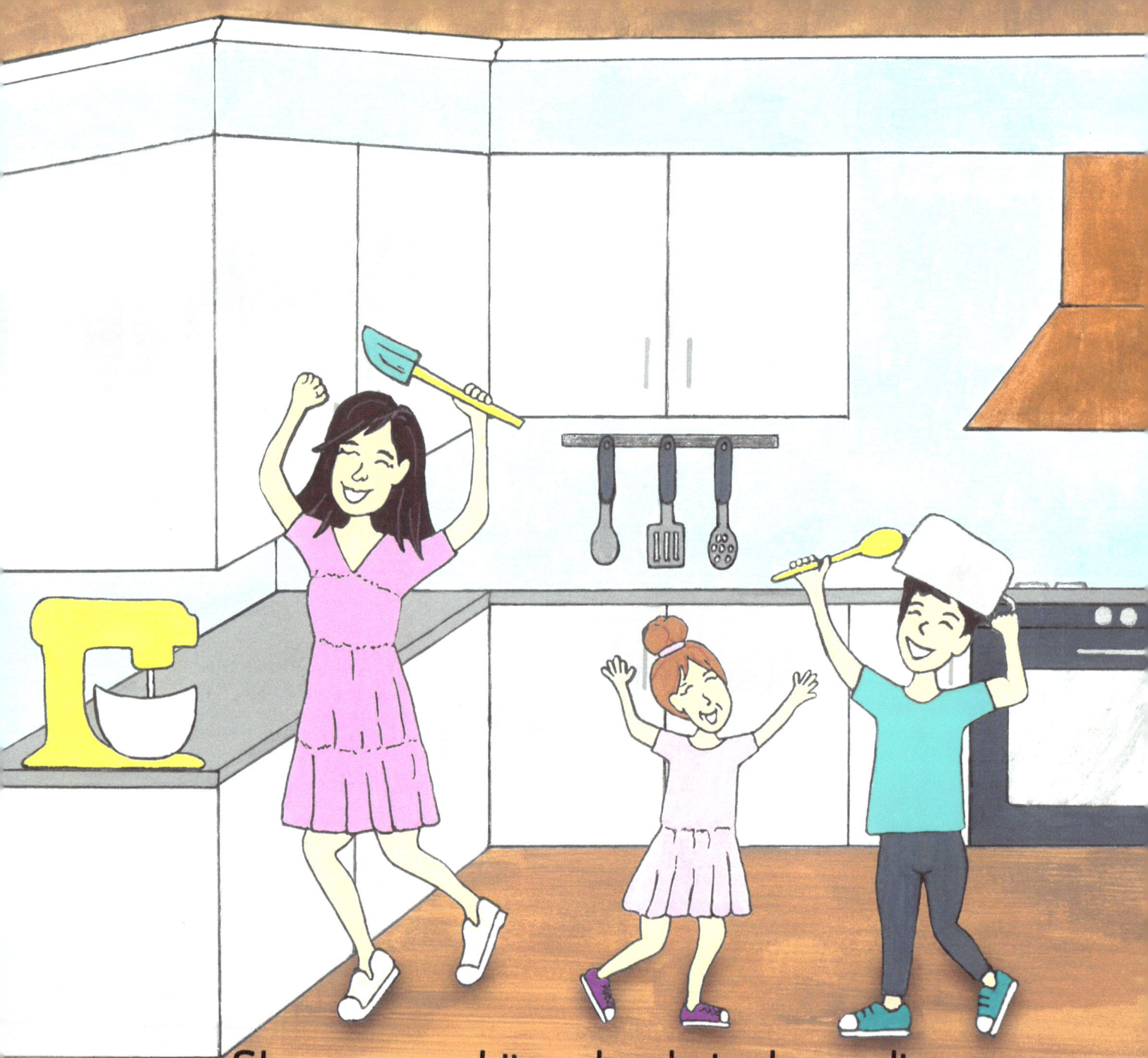

She sang while she baked goodies,
and we danced around the kitchen.

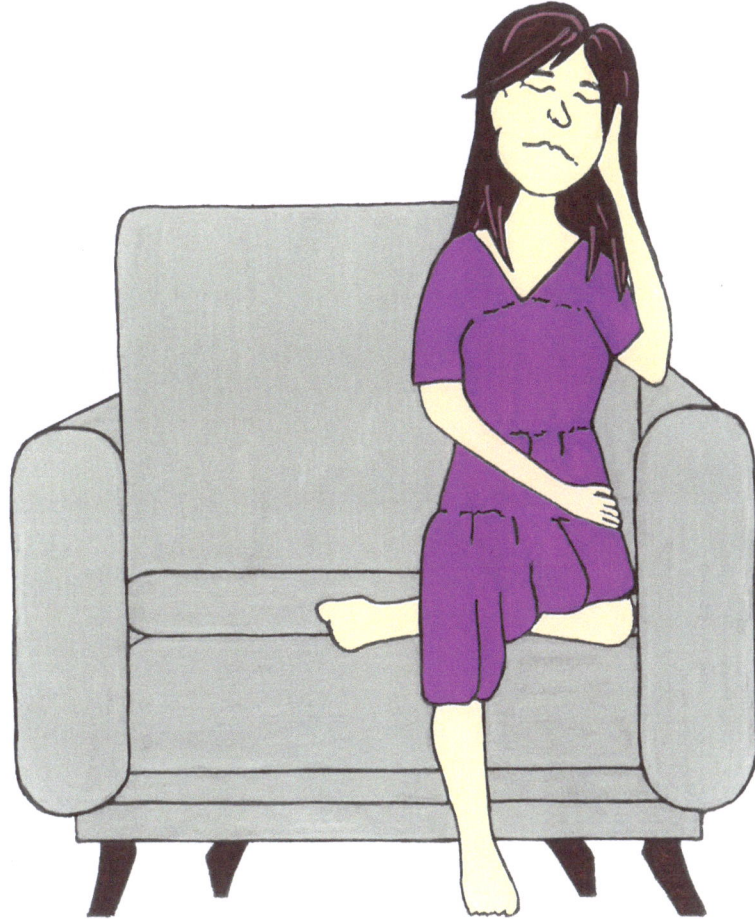

Now, singing and dancing make her tired.

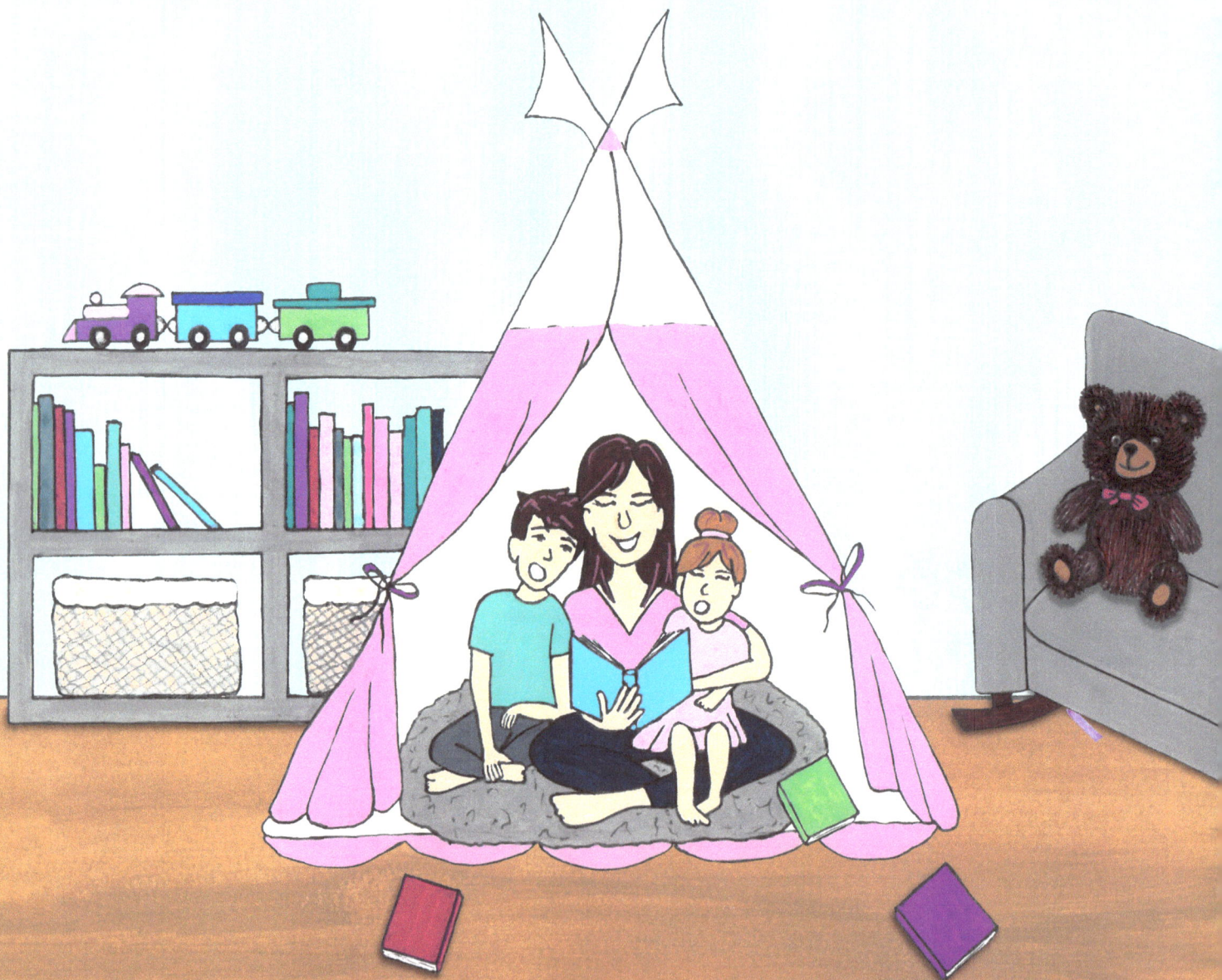

Mommy used to read books to Brother and me.

Now, Brother reads to Mommy and me.

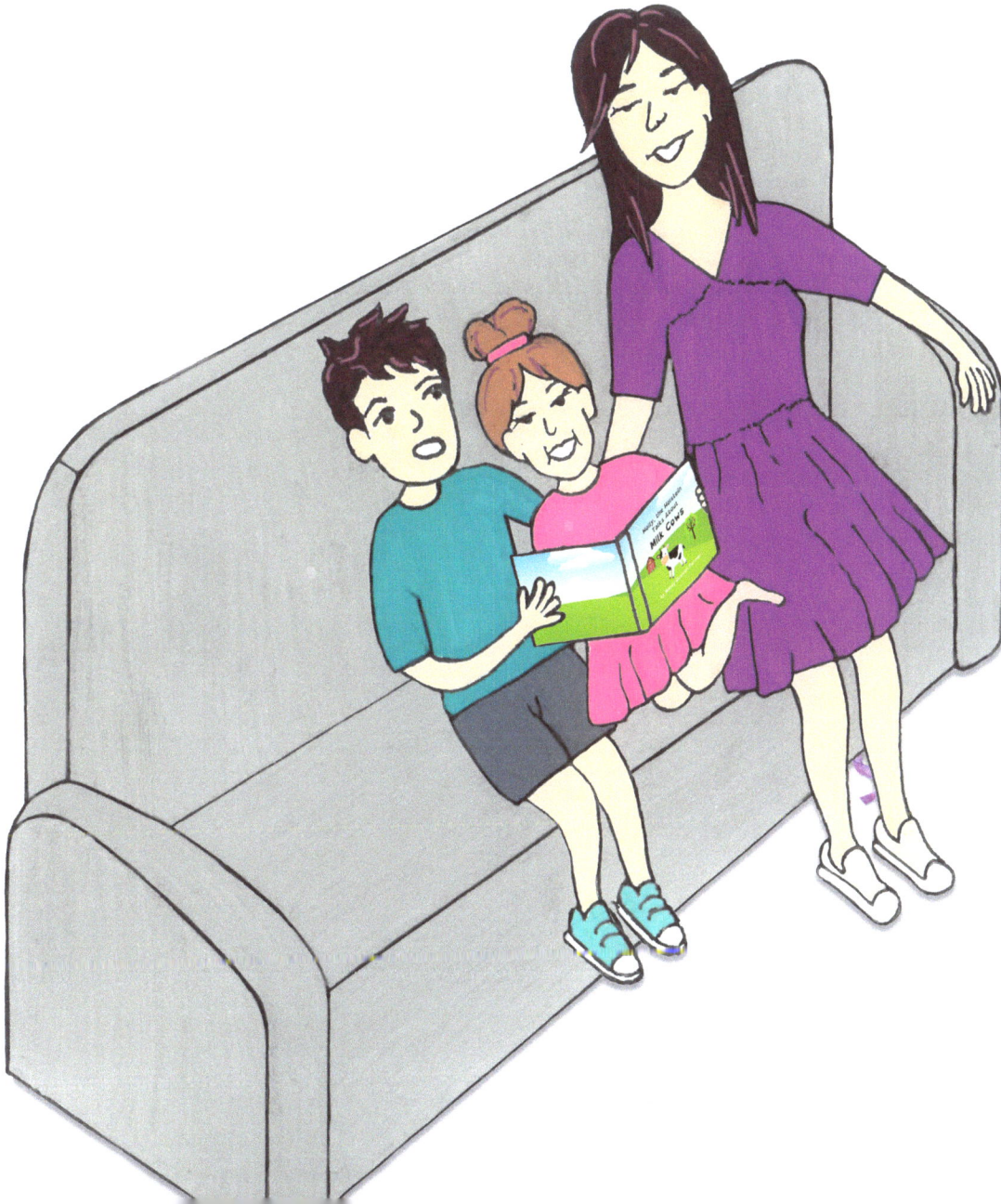

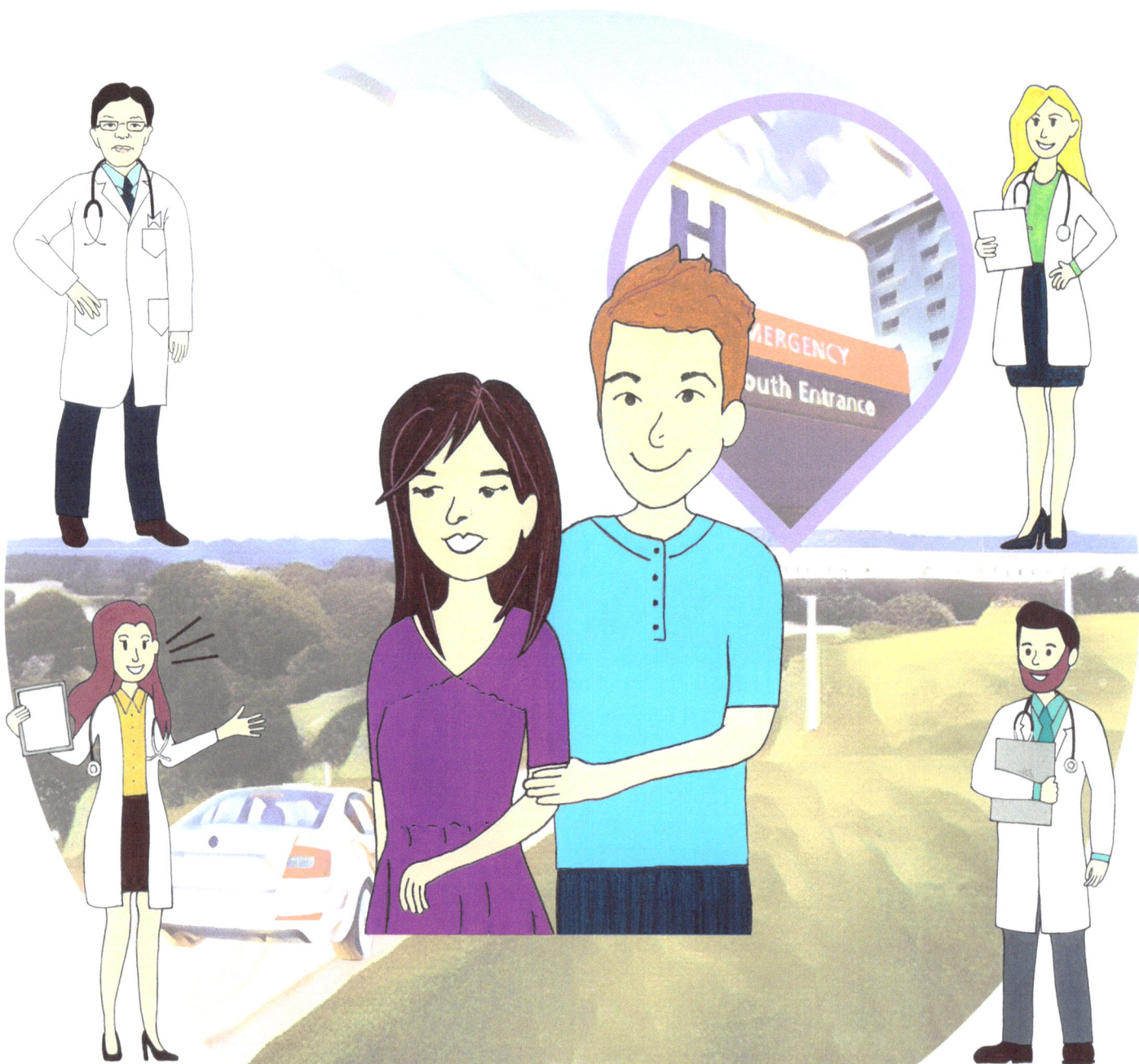

Daddy has been taking her to see lots of doctors. Some are far, far away.

One doctor said,

"You have Fiber - my - Ouch-a"

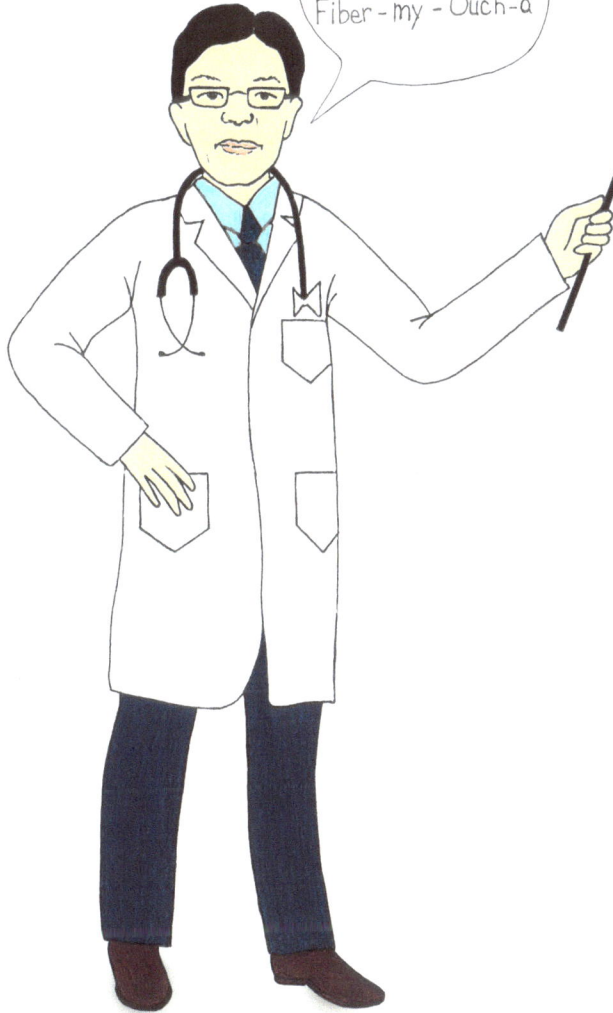

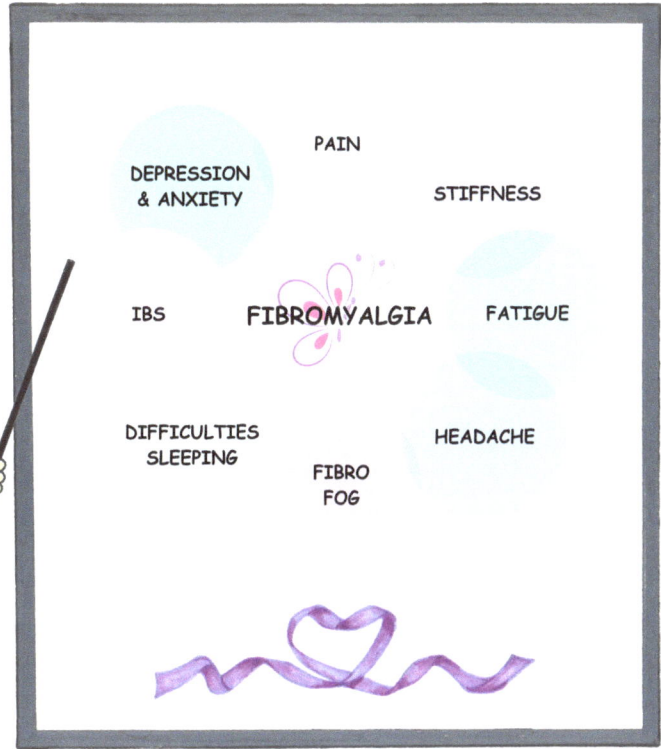

PAIN

DEPRESSION & ANXIETY

STIFFNESS

IBS

FIBROMYALGIA

FATIGUE

DIFFICULTIES SLEEPING

HEADACHE

FIBRO FOG

Fiber-my-Ouch-a means she hurts all over.

It's hard to think

I never know when my energy will be gone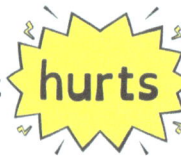

It 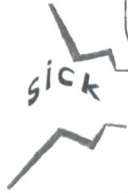 hurts to touch my arms

My tummy feels sick

My joints are stiff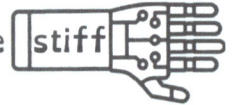

I 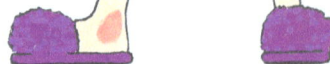 bruise easy

The doctor gave her some medicine.
It helps a little.

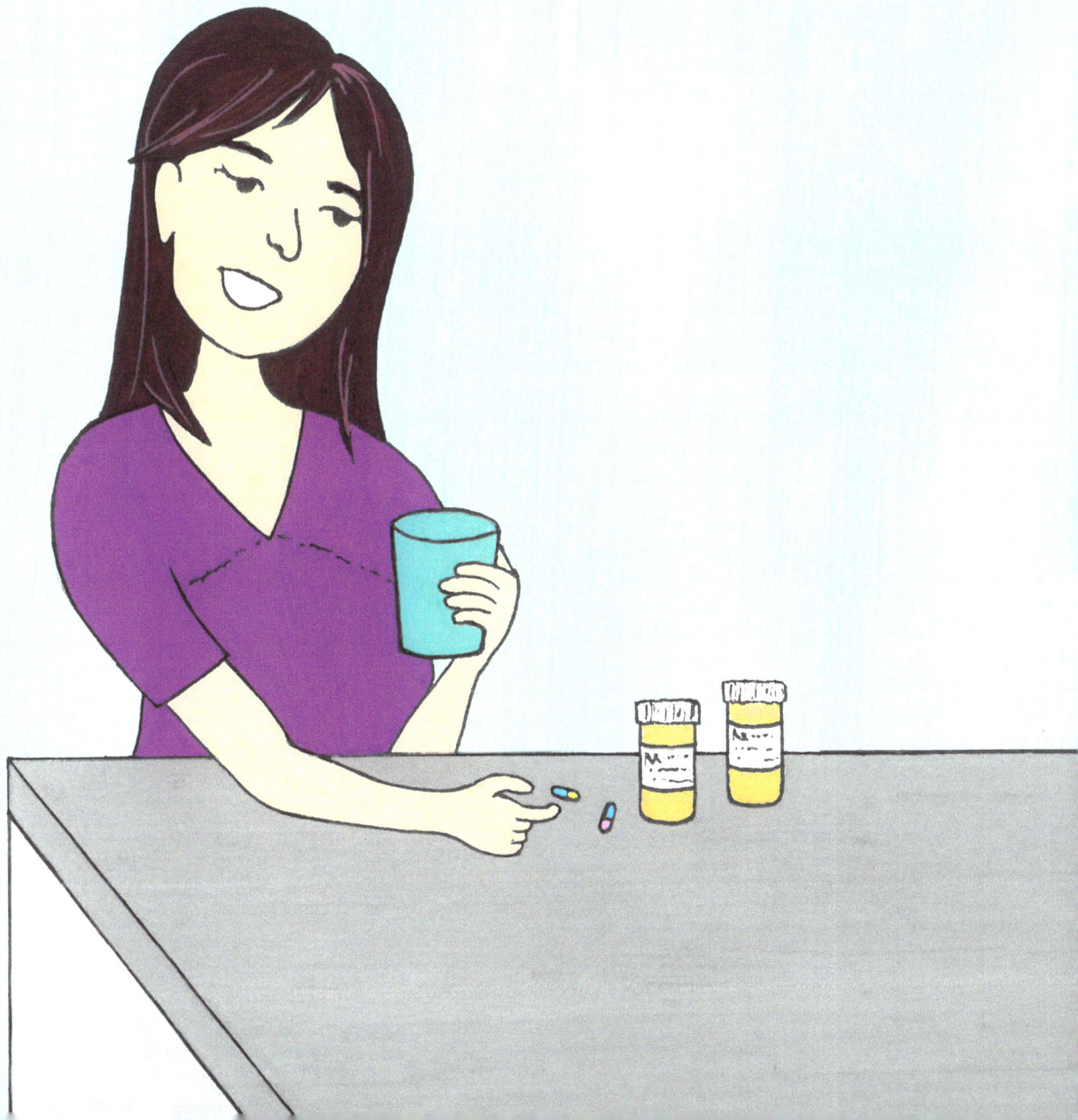

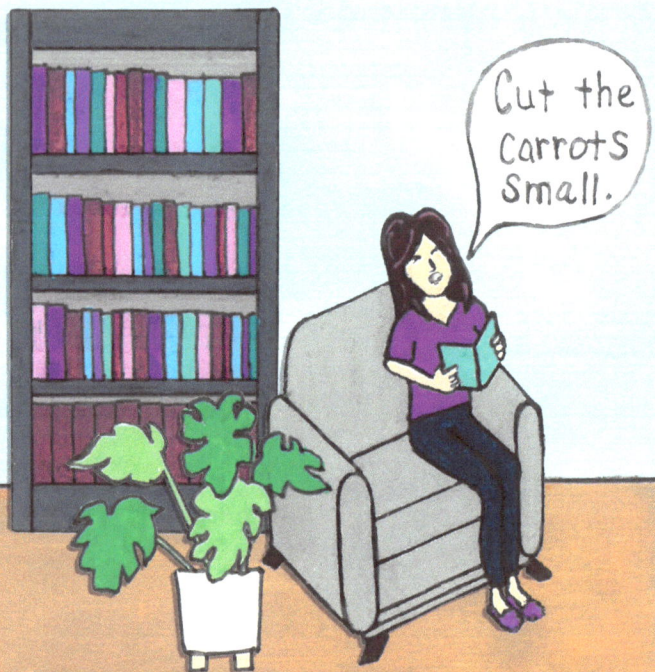

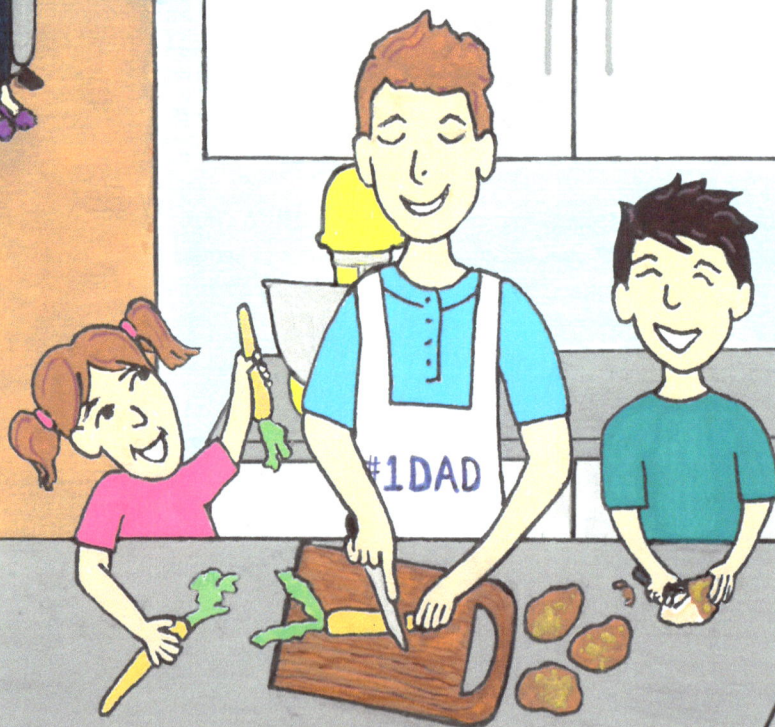

Now, we help Daddy fix supper.
Mommy sits nearby.

Sometimes, friends bring us supper.

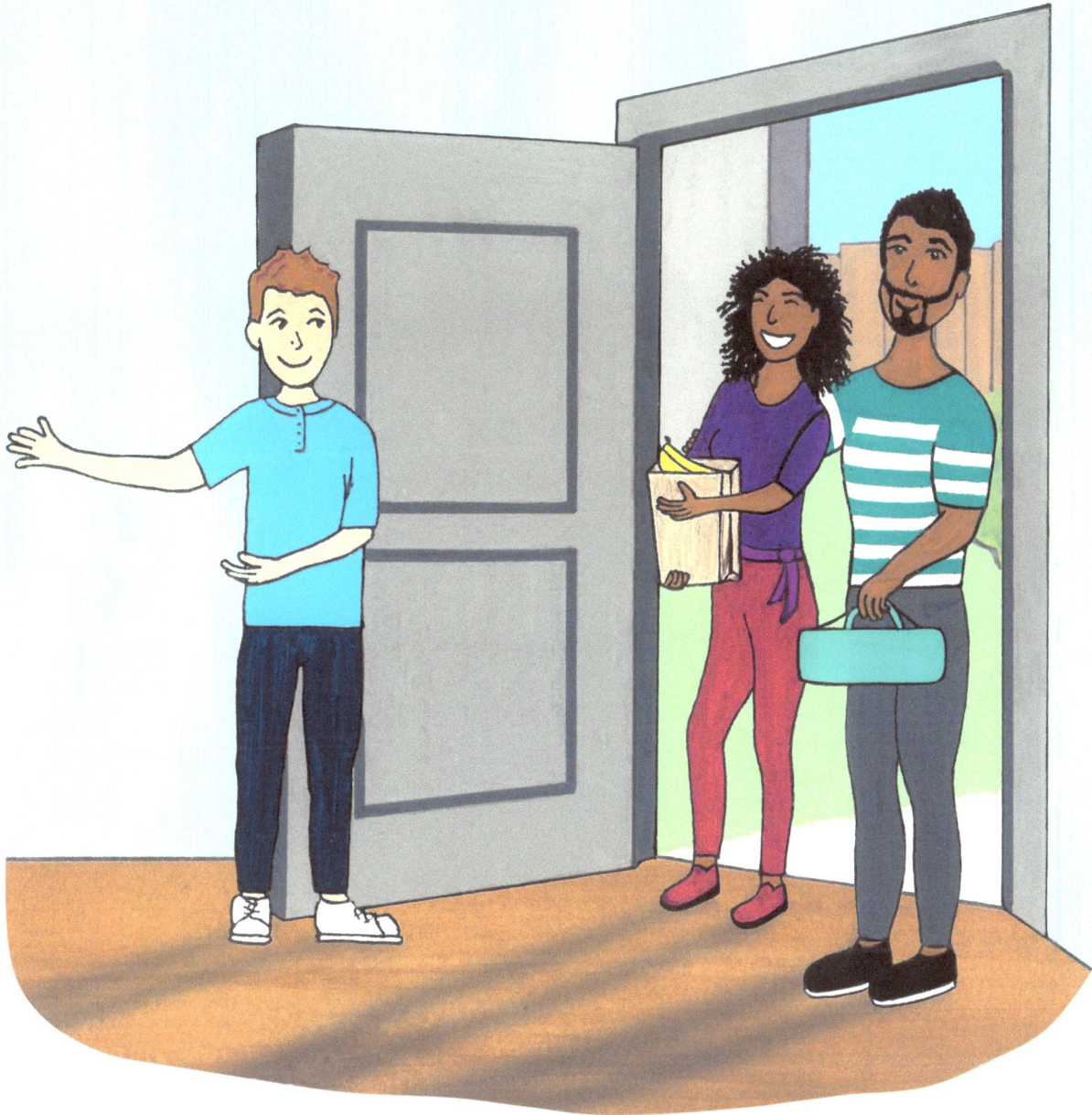

When we get scared or sad, Mommy listens and helps us find things to be thankful for.

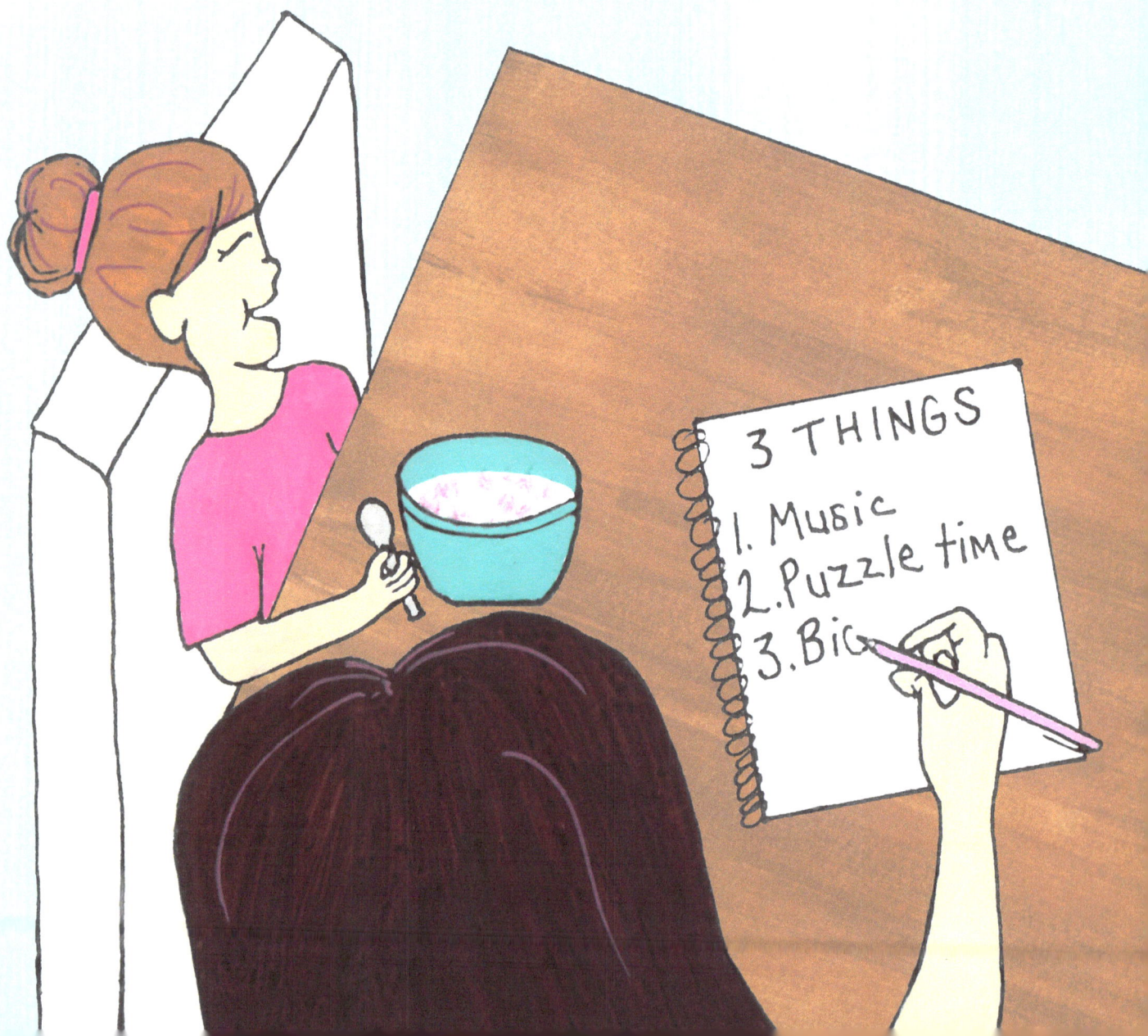

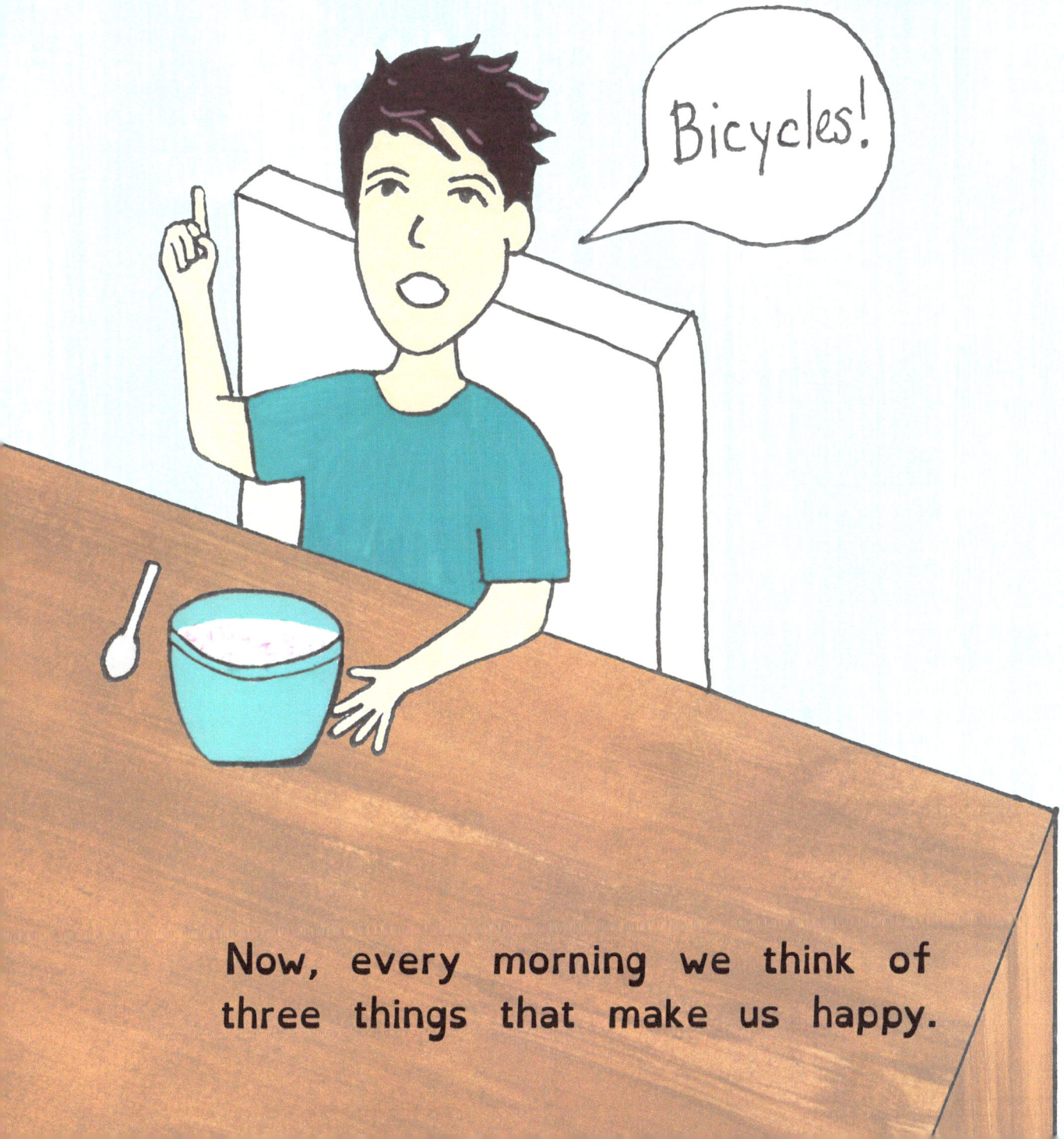

Now, every morning we think of three things that make us happy.

When Mommy has a good day,
we go outside to play.

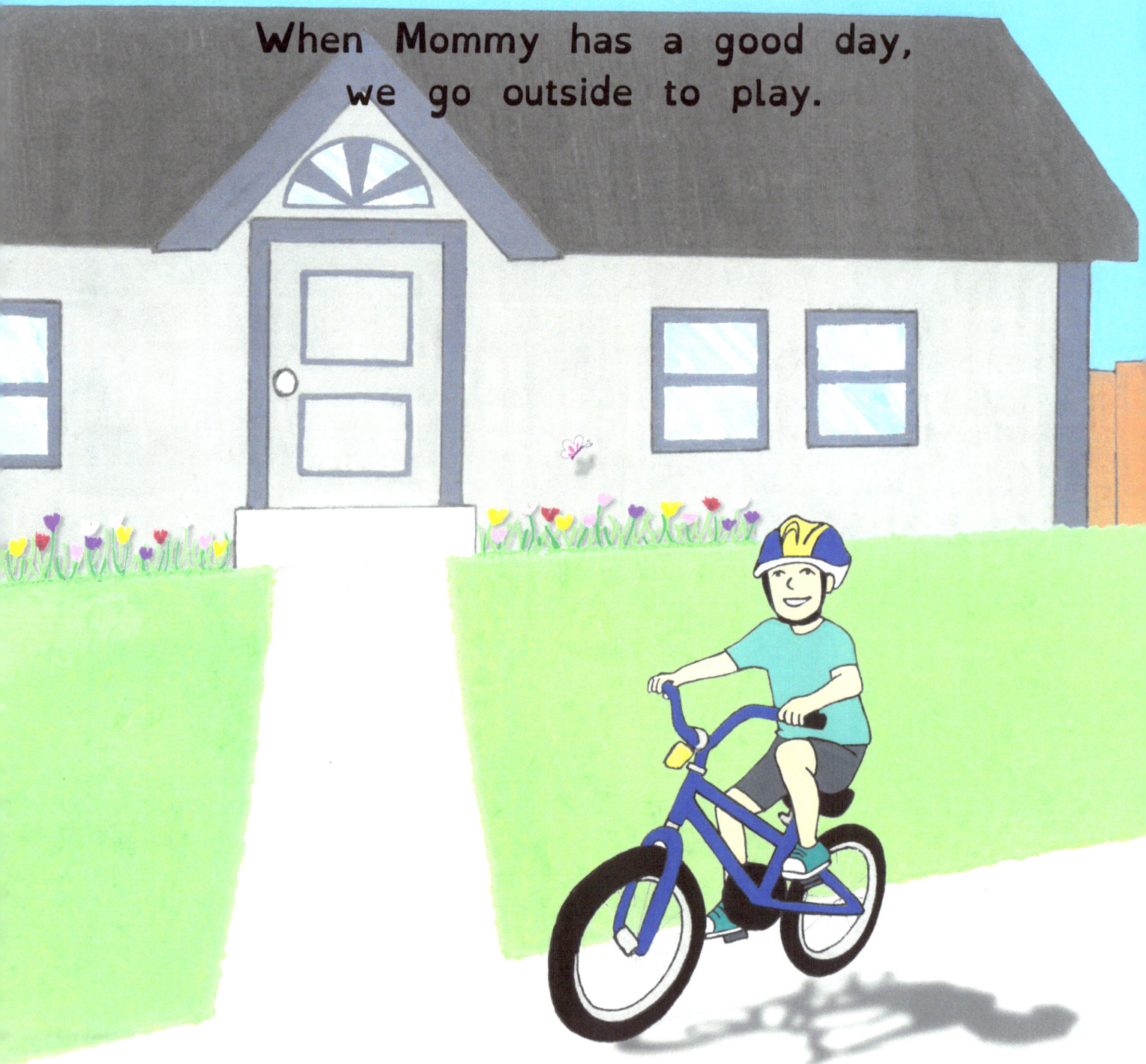

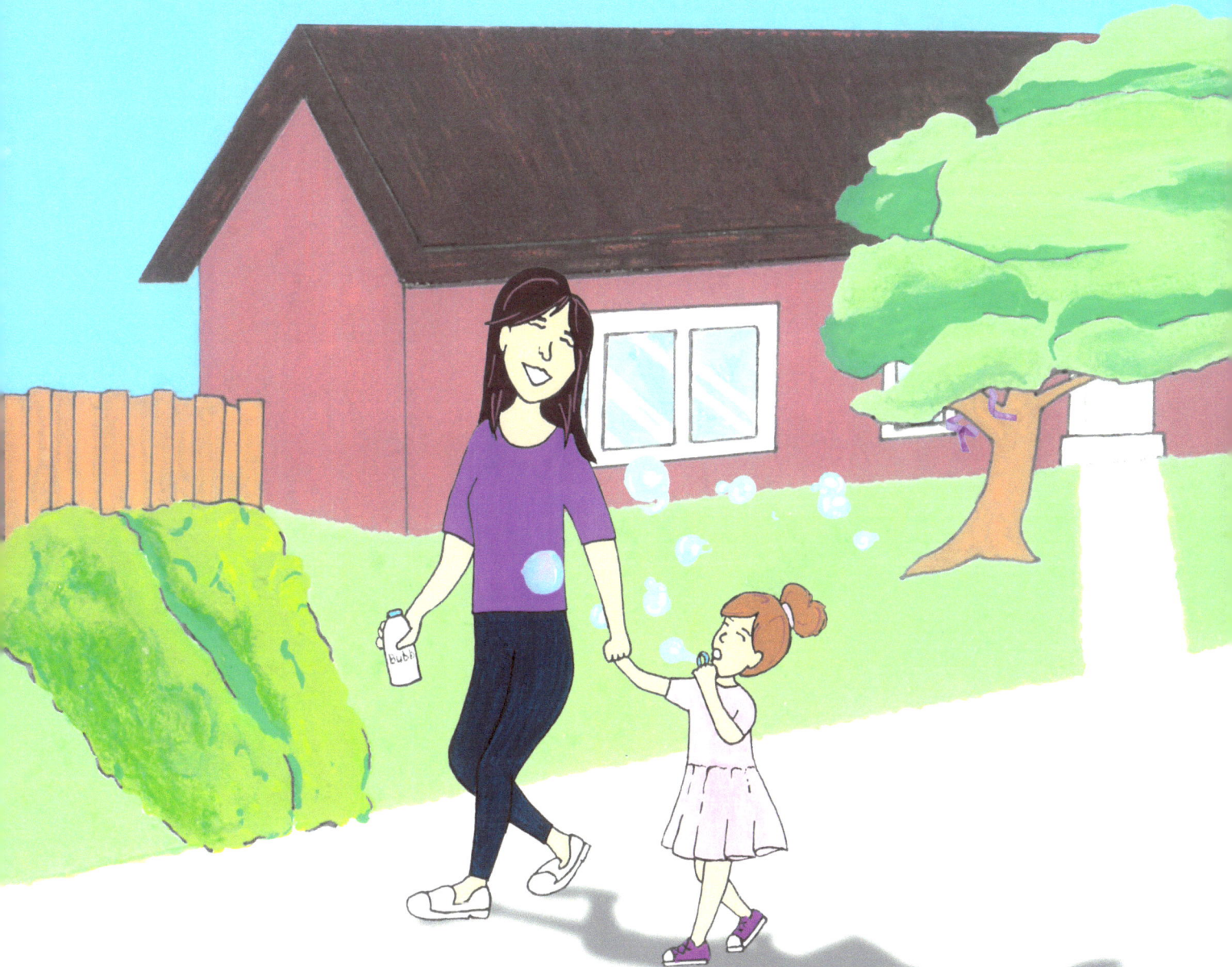

Sometimes, we take a
walk while Brother rides his bike.

On **REALLY** good days, she makes a few cookies with dough bought from a store.

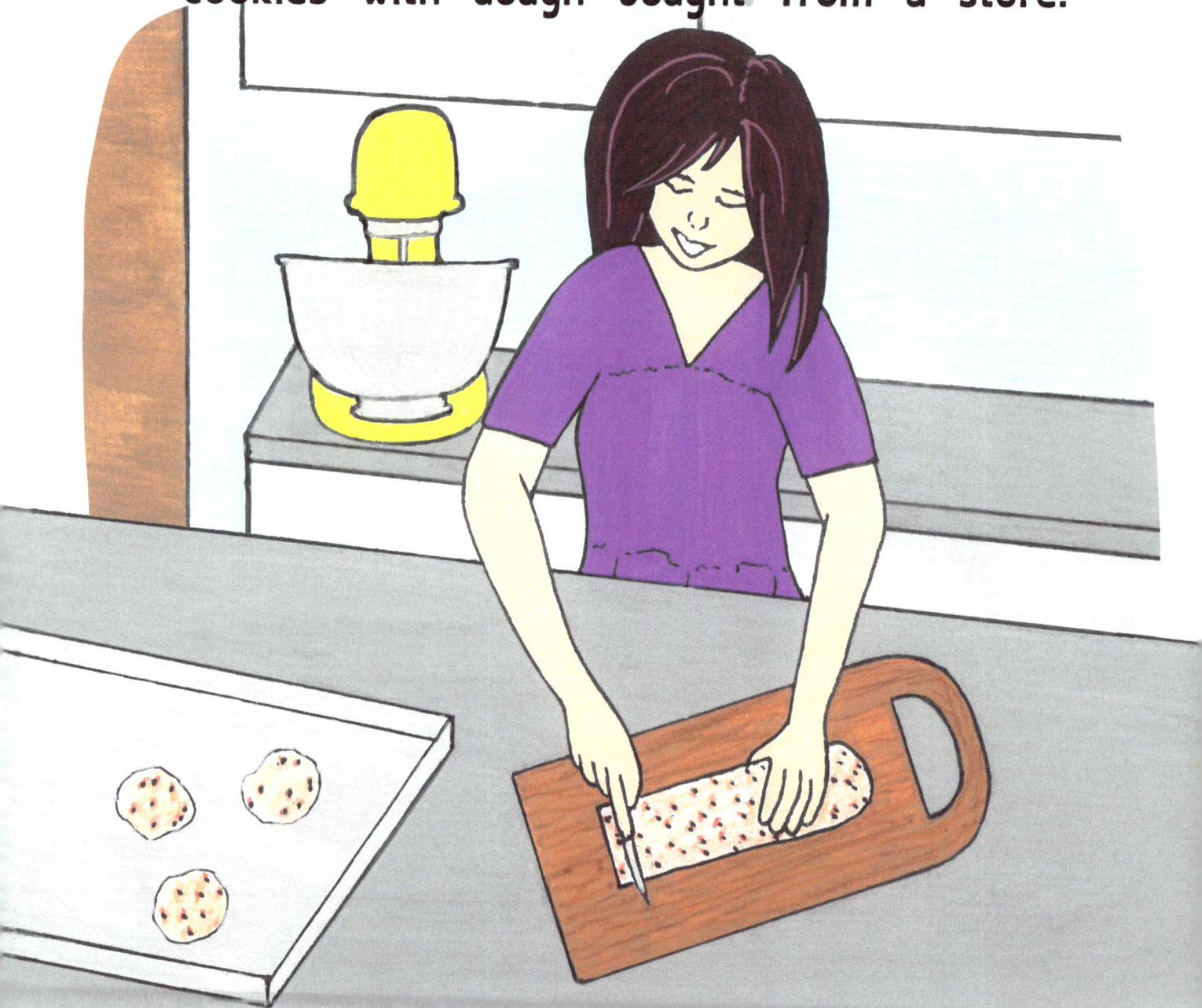

They are still yummy, since Mommy made them.

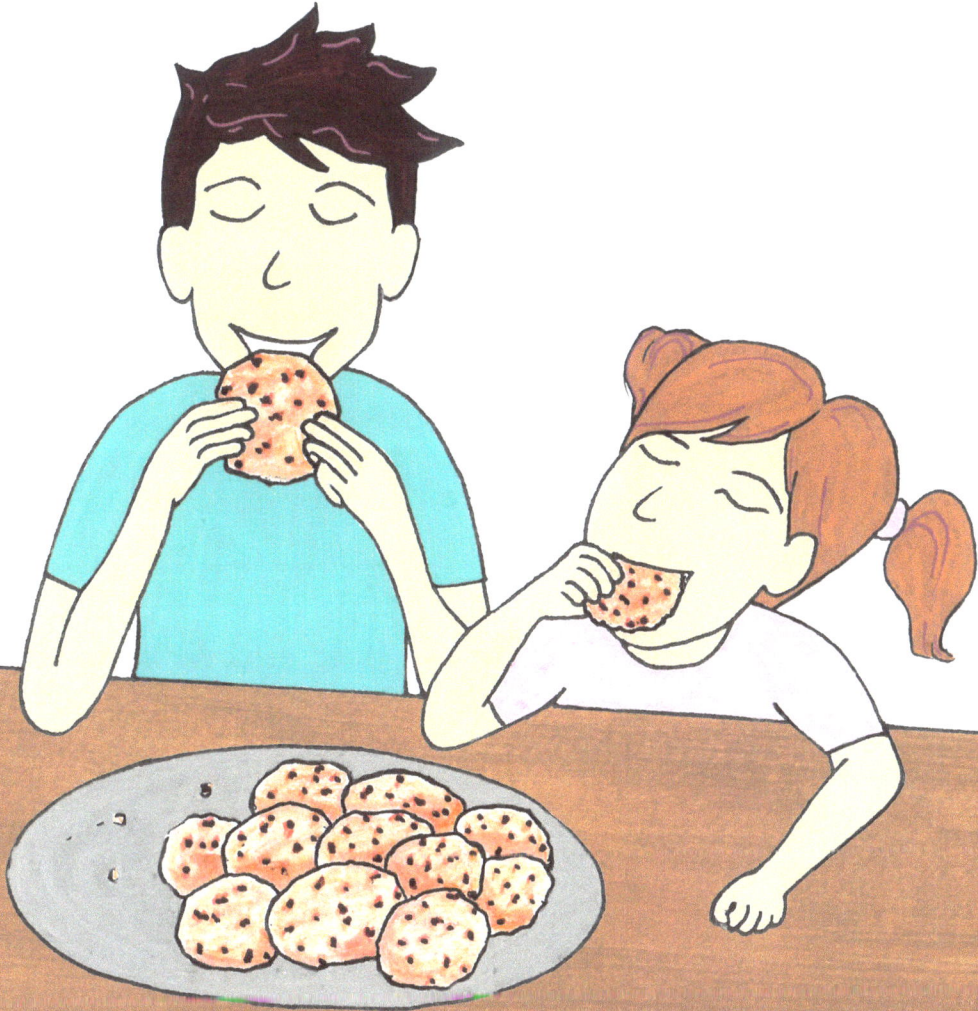

On not-so-good days, Mommy sits in the living room, and we do a show.

Brother tells us his *silly jokes.*

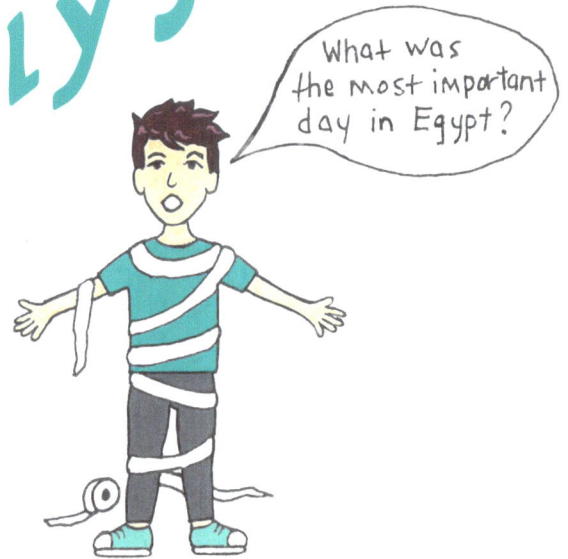

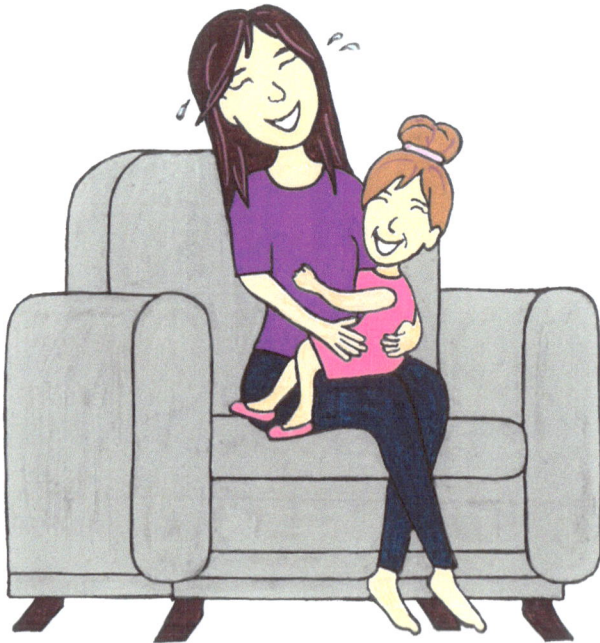

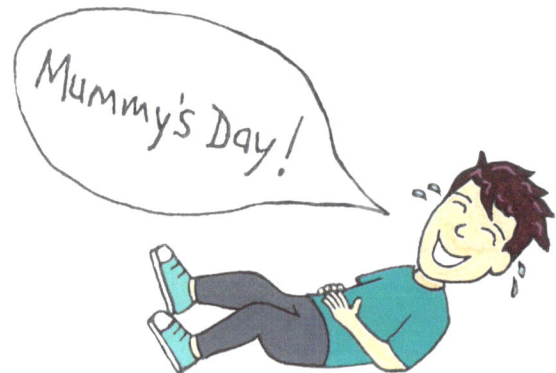

What was the most important day in Egypt?

Mummy's Day!

I sing and dance.

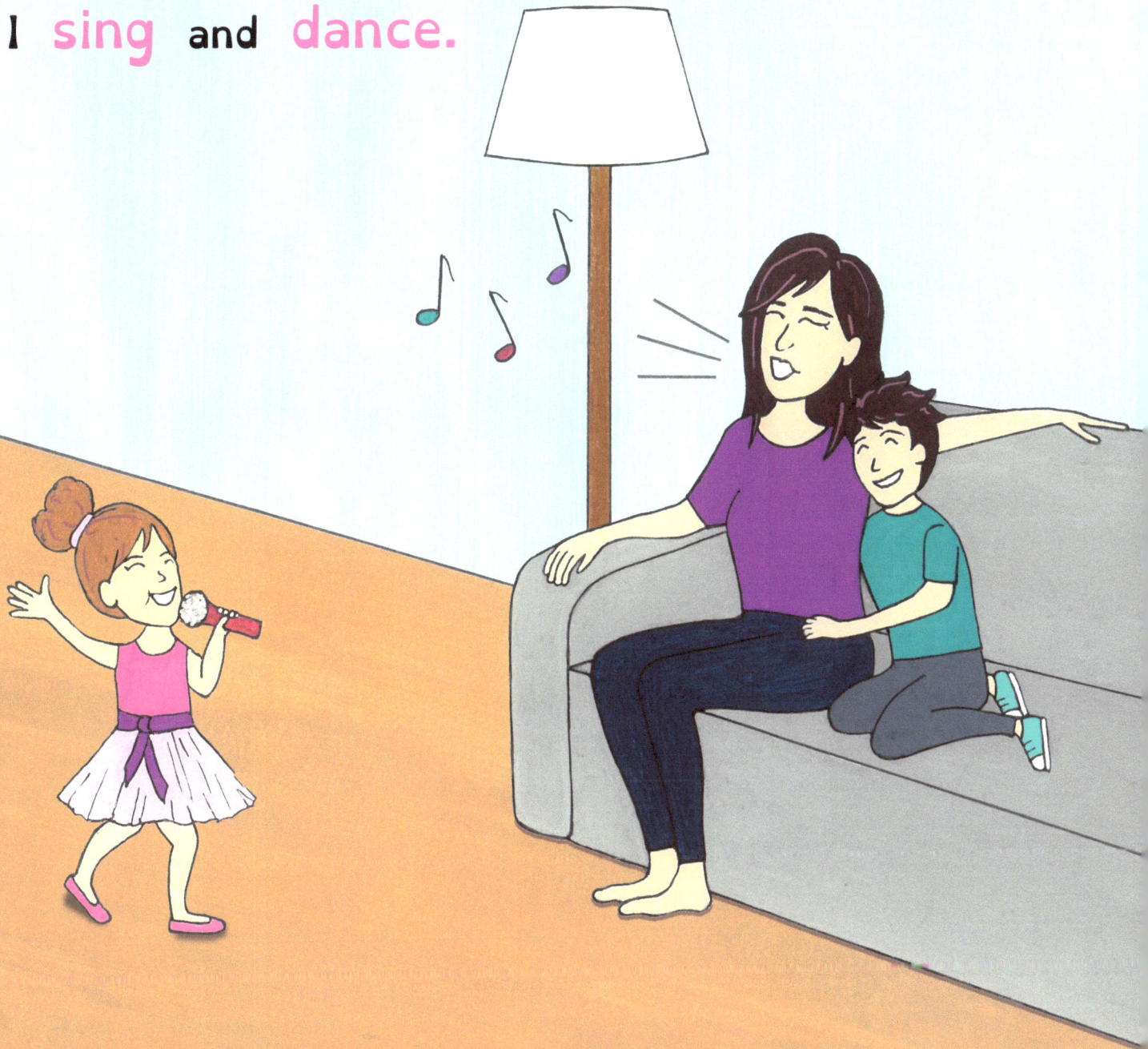

Some days, Mommy stays in bed - we climb into bed with her.

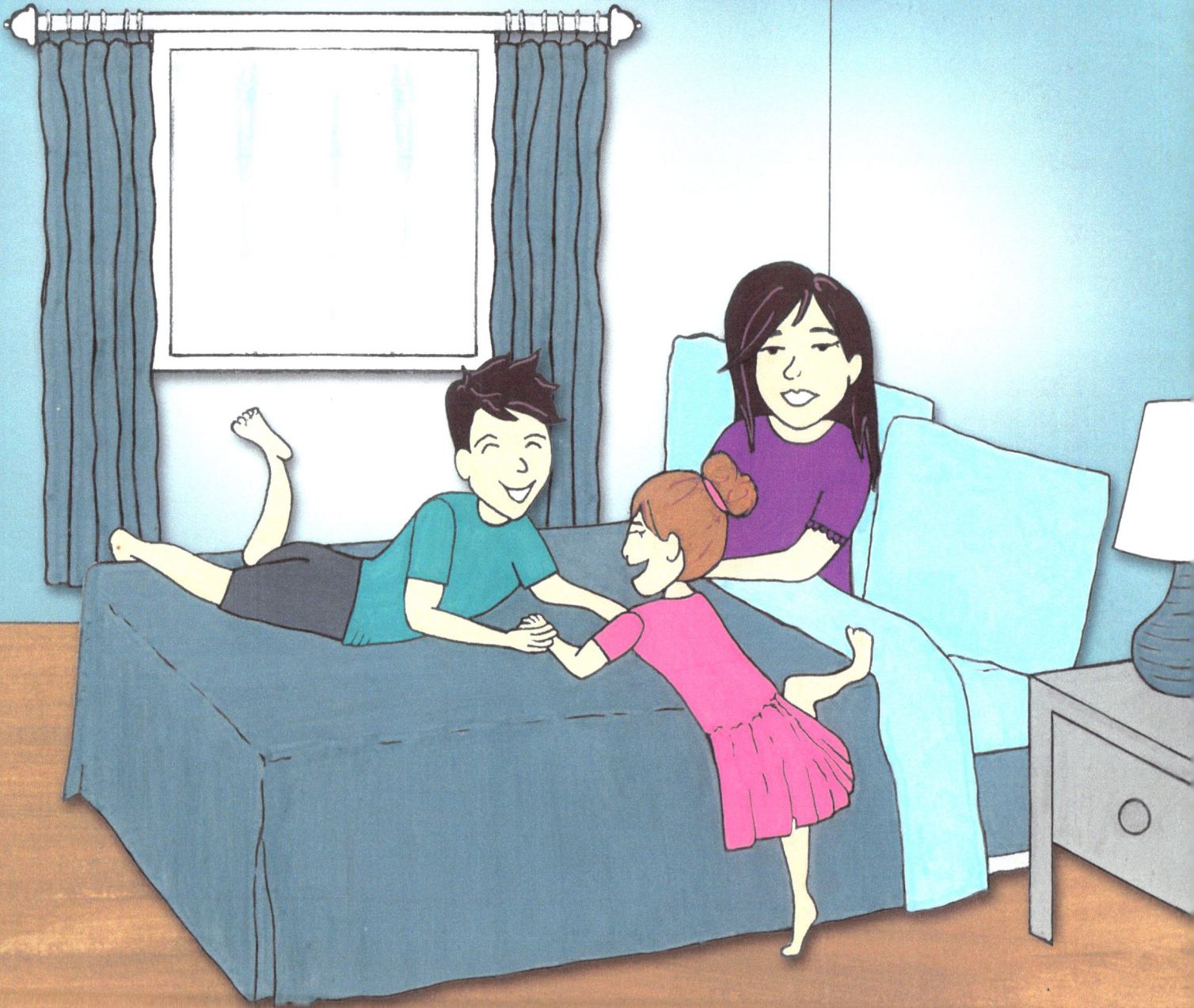

Those are some of my favorite days.

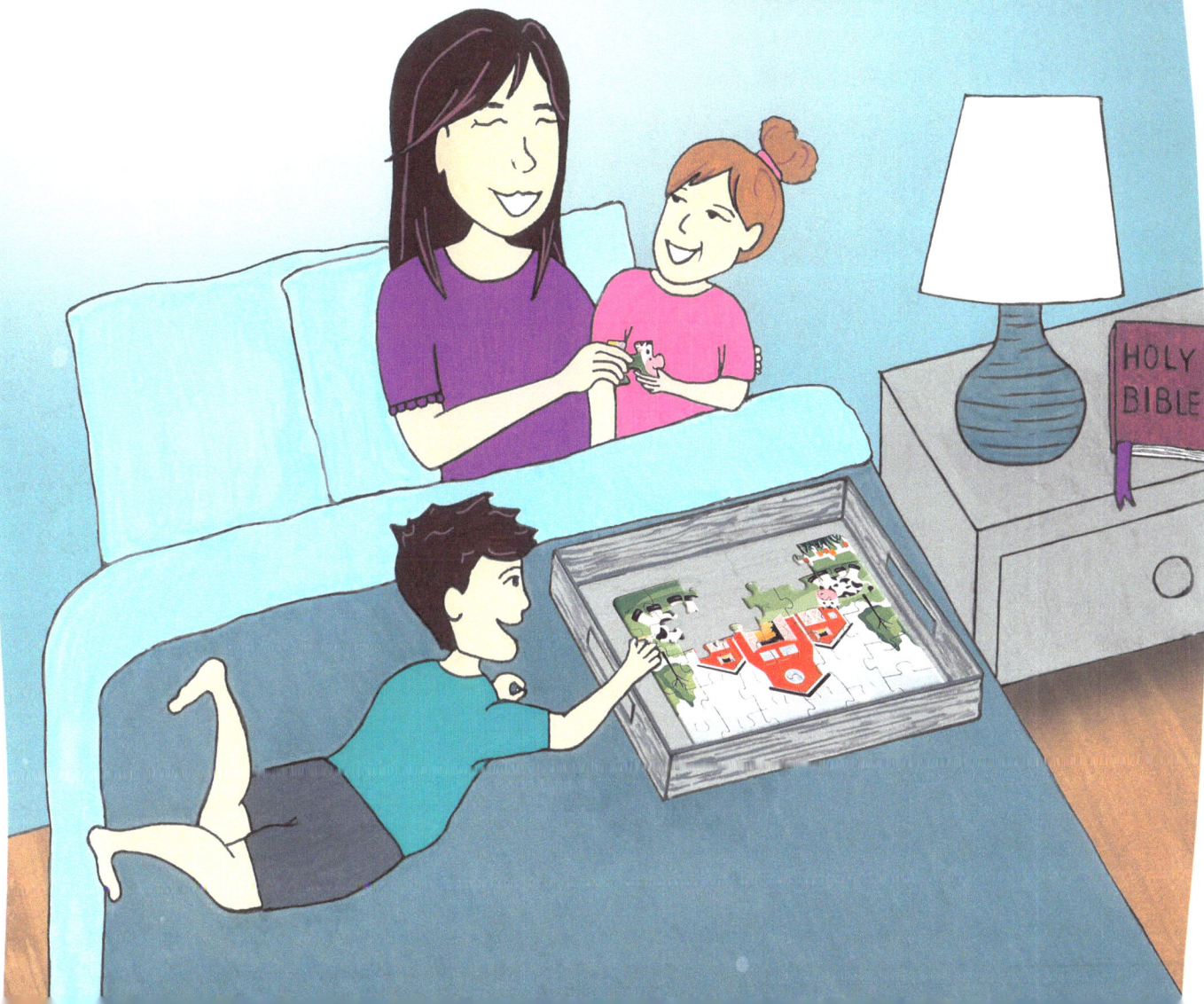

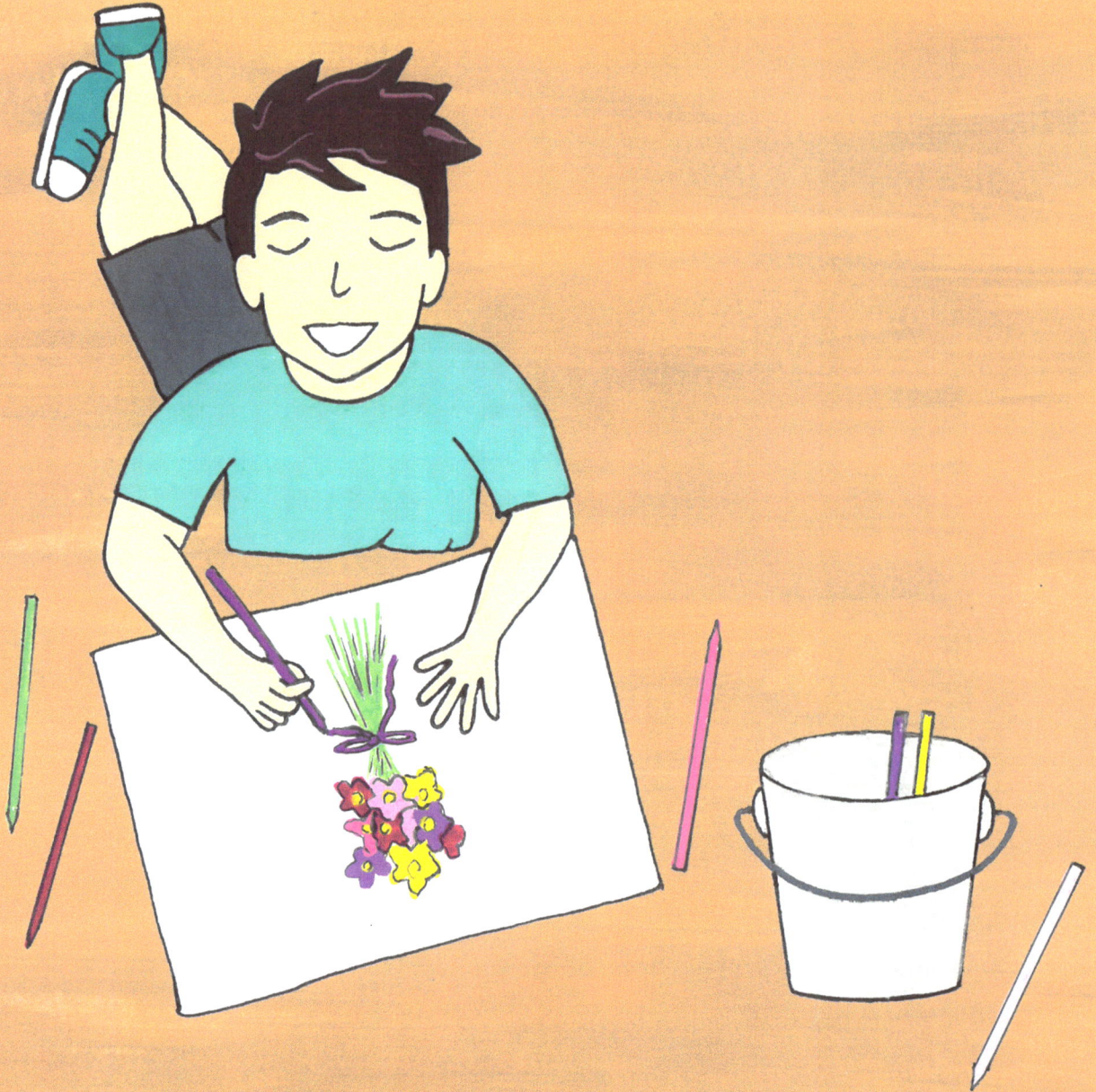

We love our Mommy.

She is still the best mommy ever...

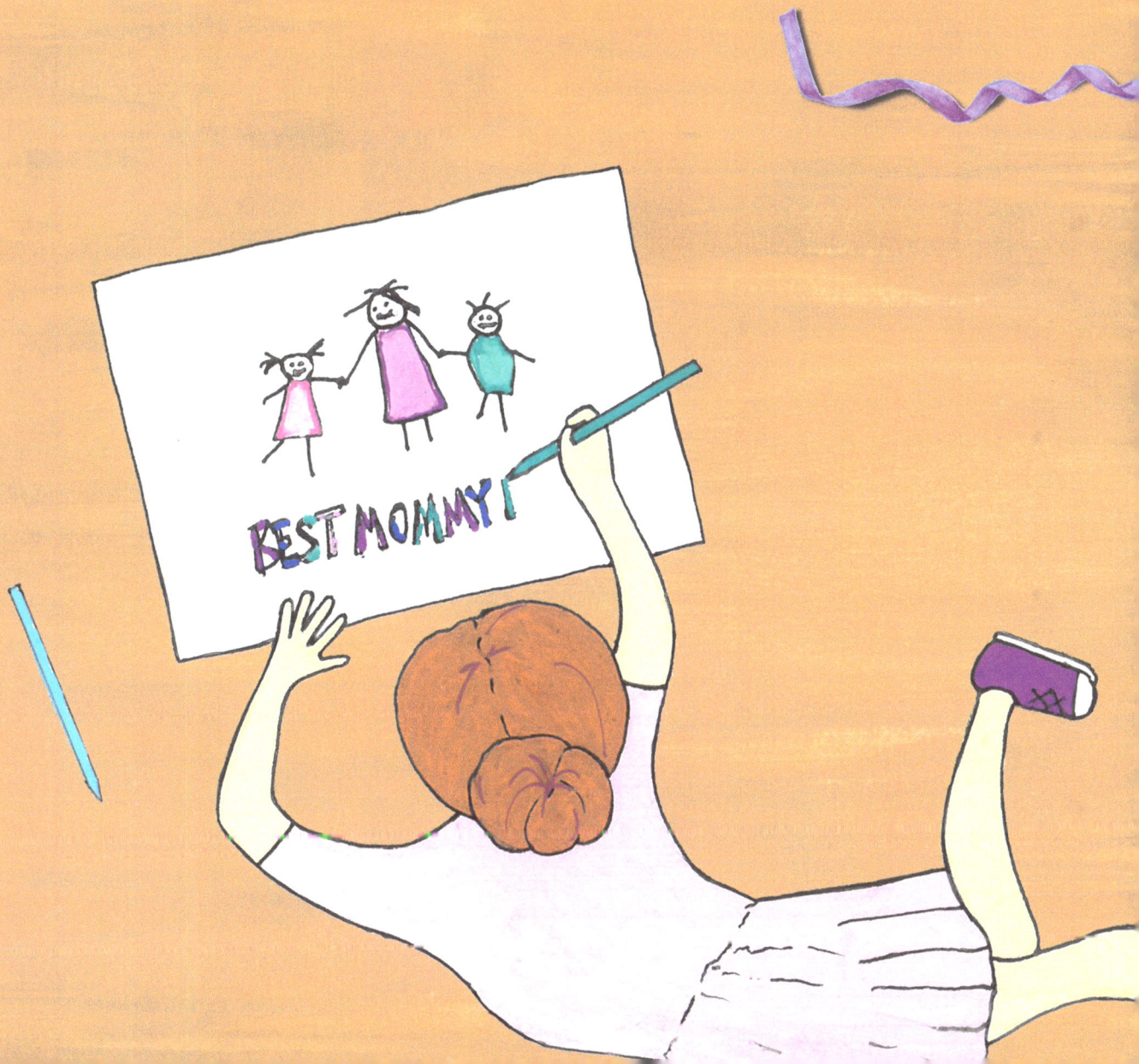

She just needs soft hugs.

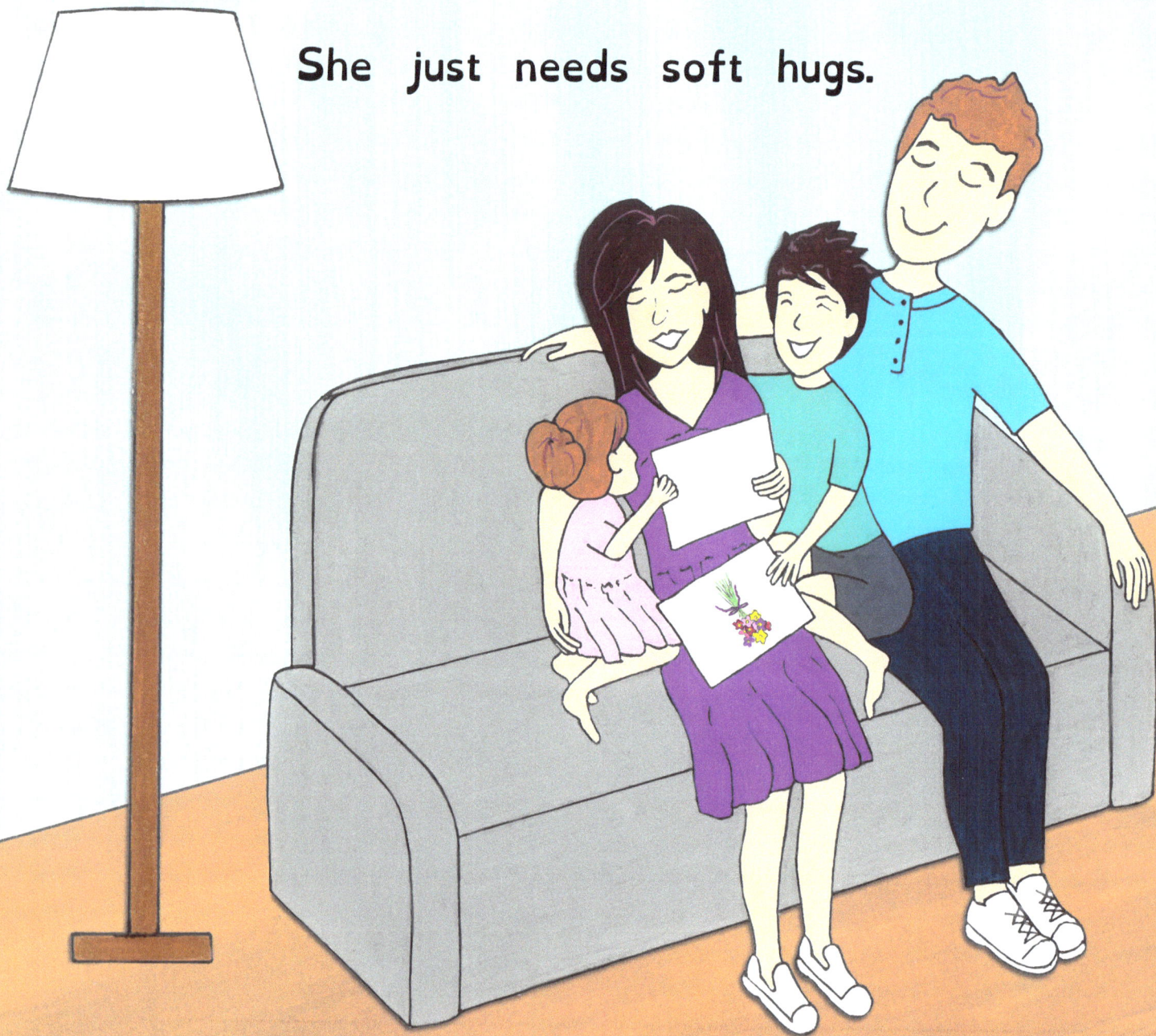

Continue the Conversation

- Q & A with your family
- Did you find **18** purple ribbons?
- Meet Mandy
- What Mandy is up to next

Turn the page for more!

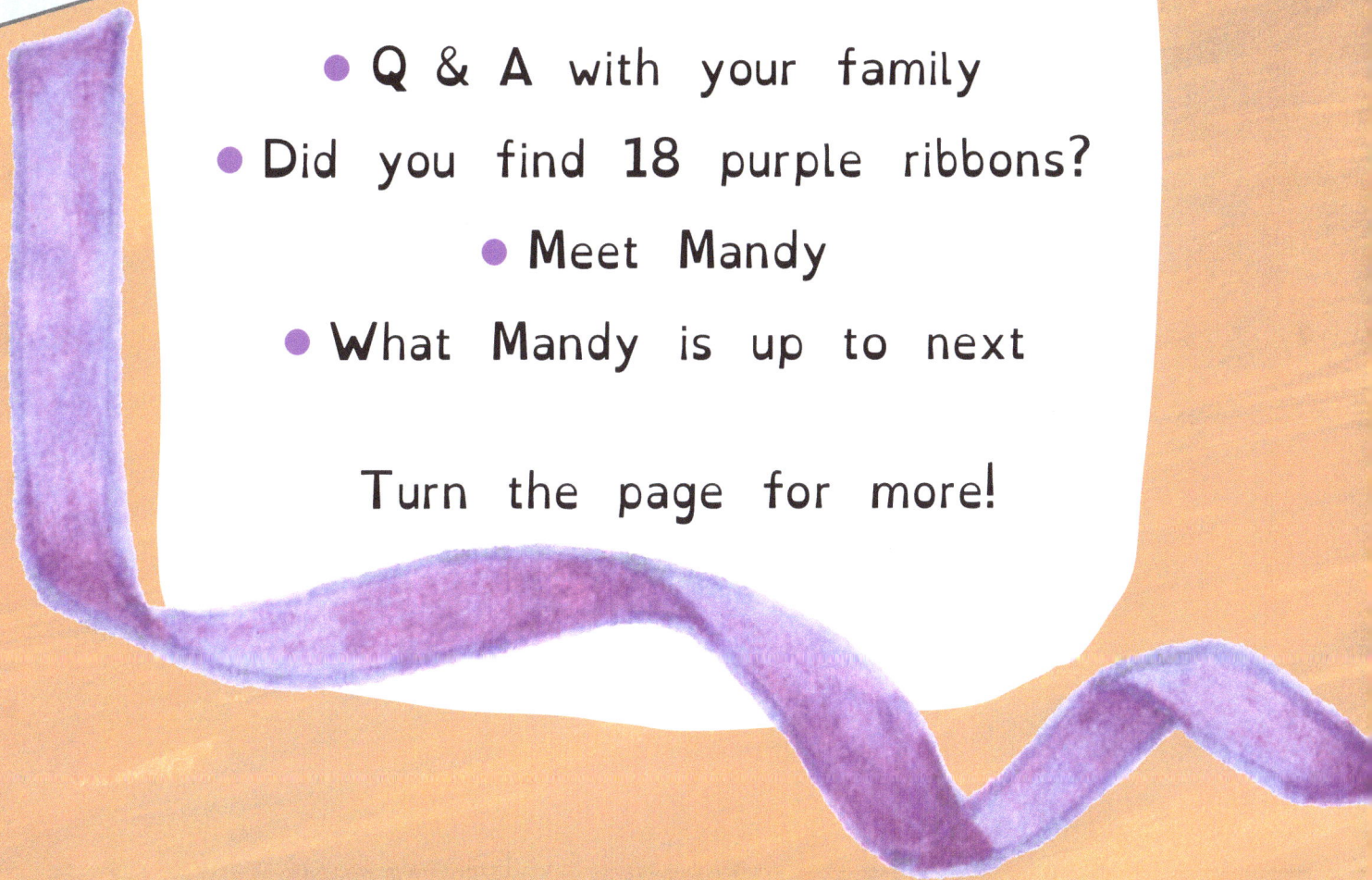

Ribbon Hunt Checklist

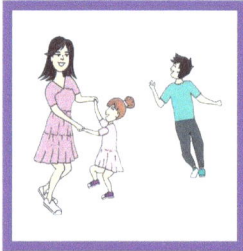

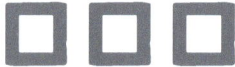

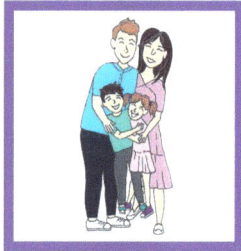

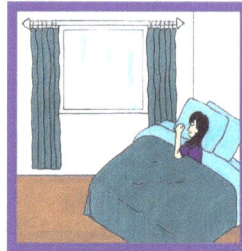

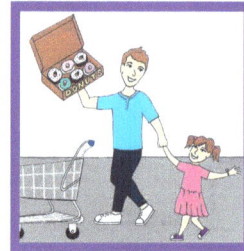

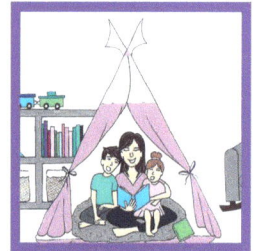

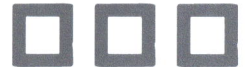

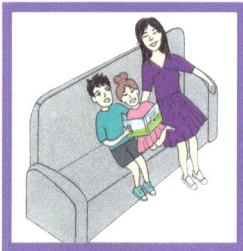

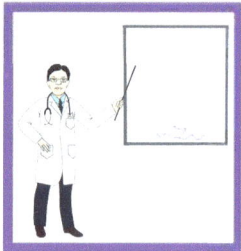

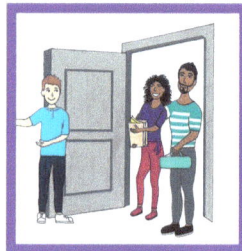

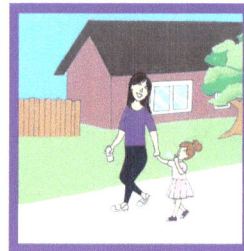

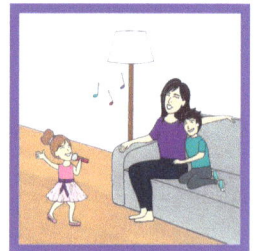

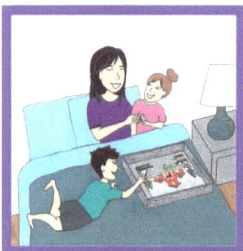

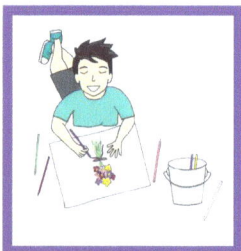

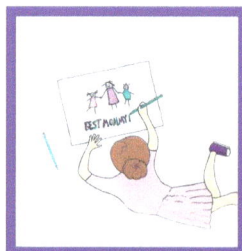

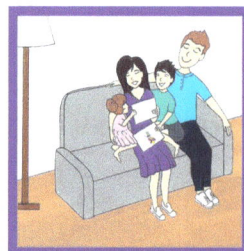

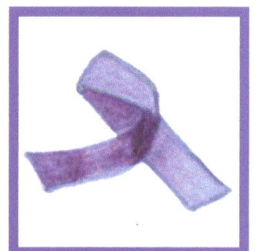

Spy purple ribbons outside your home!

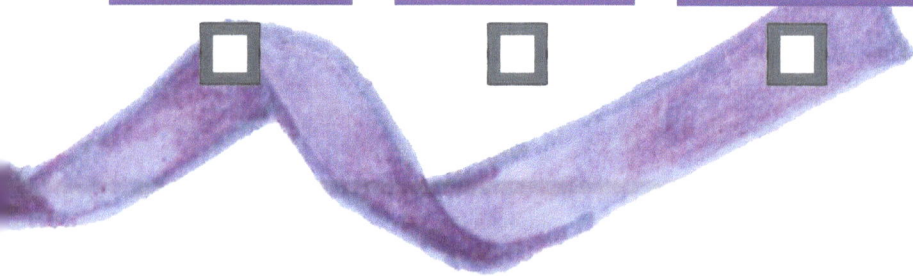

Let's Talk Fibromyalgia

1) Soft Hugs don't have to be actual hugs. It can be any act of kindness. In this book, what did the children do for their Mommy? Can you think of kind acts to help your mommy?

2) Is there anything that scares you about Mommy's illness?

3) Have you talked with anyone about your feelings since Mommy got sick? How did you feel after that?

4) What things do you miss or wish you could do with Mommy?

5) Are there times when you feel angry or mad about Mommy being sick? Let's talk about that.

6) What are some things you can do when you are worried or upset about Mommy?

7) Is there anything you want to tell Mommy or Daddy about how you are feeling? Is there anything you need from them?

Meet the Illustrator

🌐 www.melissagpickens.com

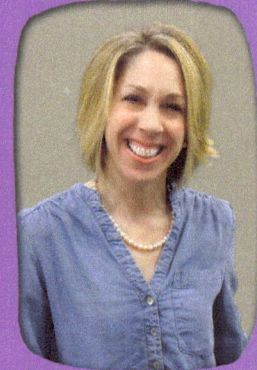

✉️ melissa@melissagpickens.com

📷 @melissagpickens

📌 @melissagpickens

f @melissagpickens

Melissa G. Pickens has been illustrating the world around her since she was old enough to hold a crayon. She and her husband reside in the amicable state of Georgia with their Micro Bernedoodle pup. Surprised by multiple chronic illnesses in midlife that challenged the trajectory of their empty nest, she was inspired to illustrate this children's book by the love her husband and 4 (now adult) kids show her as they walk this difficult terrain together. Melissa's twin grandchildren keep her wonder alive and color her world through their toddler view.

She is also a compassionate writer, who believes both art and words can help others bravely face their pain with God until it becomes a pearl. Learn more at the links above.

Meet the Author

Mandy Farmer served as a pastor's wife and children's minister for over **25** years; teaching, singing, and developing curriculum. However, in **2011**, her life took an unexpected turn, and she found herself on her back in excruciating pain. Mandy and her husband retired in **2016** and moved to Savannah, Georgia near their **4** adult children.

Mandy's farm heritage led her to write a picture book based on farm life. Her first self-published picture book, Holly the Holstein Talks About Milk Cows, emerged in **2022**.

She started blogging about her journey with pain and her faith and saw a need within the family context for understanding chronic illness. Out of this burning awareness emerged "Soft Hugs". Follow her on www.mandyfarmer.com and receive monthly "hugs" for your journey with pain and news on her upcoming books.

@mandy_farmer_author

@mandolyn1025

Fibromyalgia is it for Real?

author@mandyfarmer.com

www.mandyfarmer.com

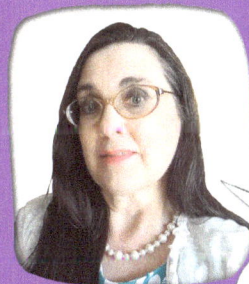

Turn the page for my other books!

Check out Mandy's other books available now!

Holly, the Holstein Talks About **Milk Cows**

. Mandy Dawson Farmer

available at **amazon**

A,B,C's Down on the Farm Coloring Book

available at **amazon**

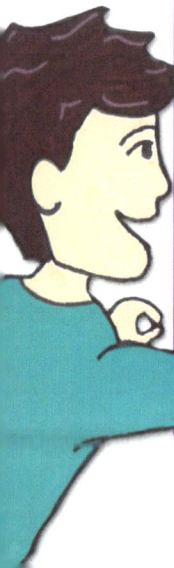

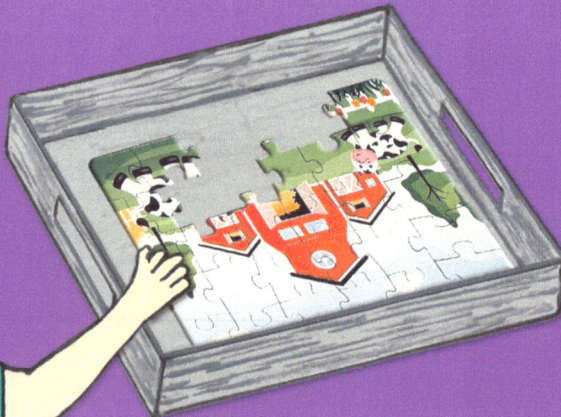

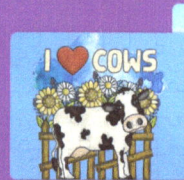

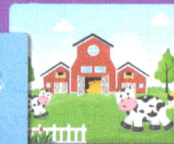

Check out my Etsy Store for puzzles, gifts, and more!

From Dissonant to Harmonious
Devotions for Your Journey with Pain

Chronic pain steals your life. It takes your health, daily life, family time, hobbies, social life, and finally, your job and home. How do we come to grips with this? How do you stop the downward spiral into depression and a long life of trials and tribulations?

Mandy found her way through the trials without losing the song in her heart. In her book of devotions, she shares moments from her story by connecting with historical and Biblical people. Studying these counterparts, she finds brief notes of encouragement. Mandy invites you to join in her journey to help ease your pain. Coming together and holding each other up makes the journey so much easier.

As a lover of music, she has arranged these devotions with a theme of music. Each devotion has these parts:

My Dissonant Tone
(a tidbit of my story)

Our Counterpoint
(a Biblical person with whom we can relate.)

The Harmonious Chords
(a teaching point drawn from both stories)

Practice, Practice, Practice
(read a Psalm & meditate on the lyrics of an old hymn)

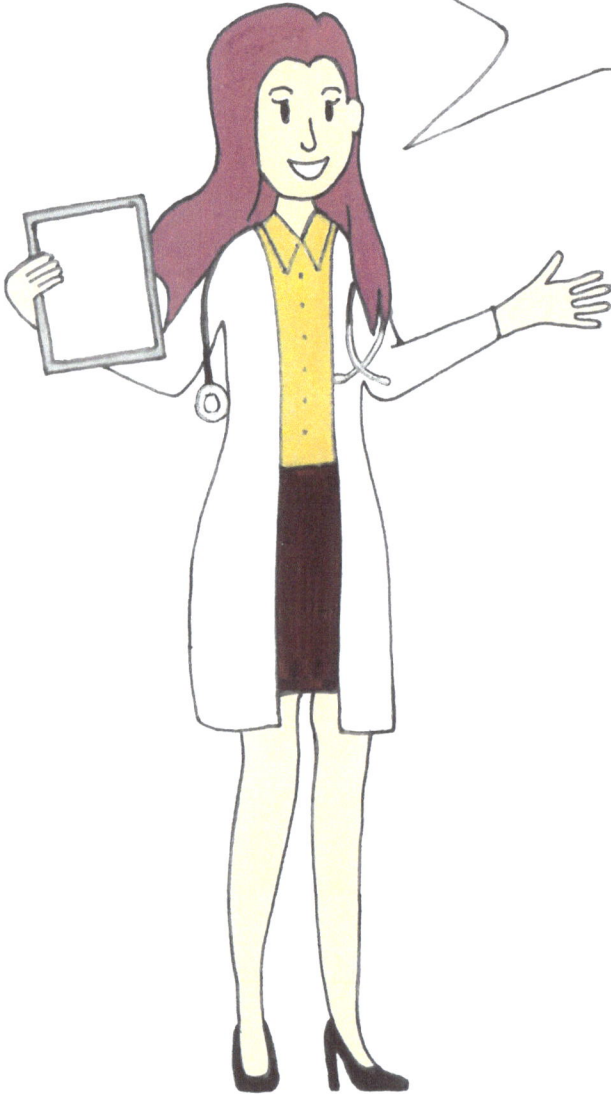

"When parents are faced with health crises, children often don't understand, and they become afraid. Soft Hugs for Mommy helps children easily understand what fibromyalgia is and how it affects their loved one, so they don't have to become worried or fearful. This is such an important book to help children understand the more invisible illnesses they encounter in others."

Dr. Michelle Bengtson
Board Certified Clinical Neuropsychologist and author of the award-winning book, Breaking Anxiety's Grip: How to Reclaim the Peace God Promises

Mandy draws from her personal experience with fibromyalgia and chronic pain. She breaks down very complicated and complex topics into child sized portions and comprehension levels. From her years of ministry and experience with chronic pain and health issues, she is a perfect person to write this book.

Tammy McDonald
Blogger, Speaker, Life Coach, Author of Shifted Vision and Conquering the Grief that stole Christmas. Connect with her at www.hopeforgrievinghearts.com

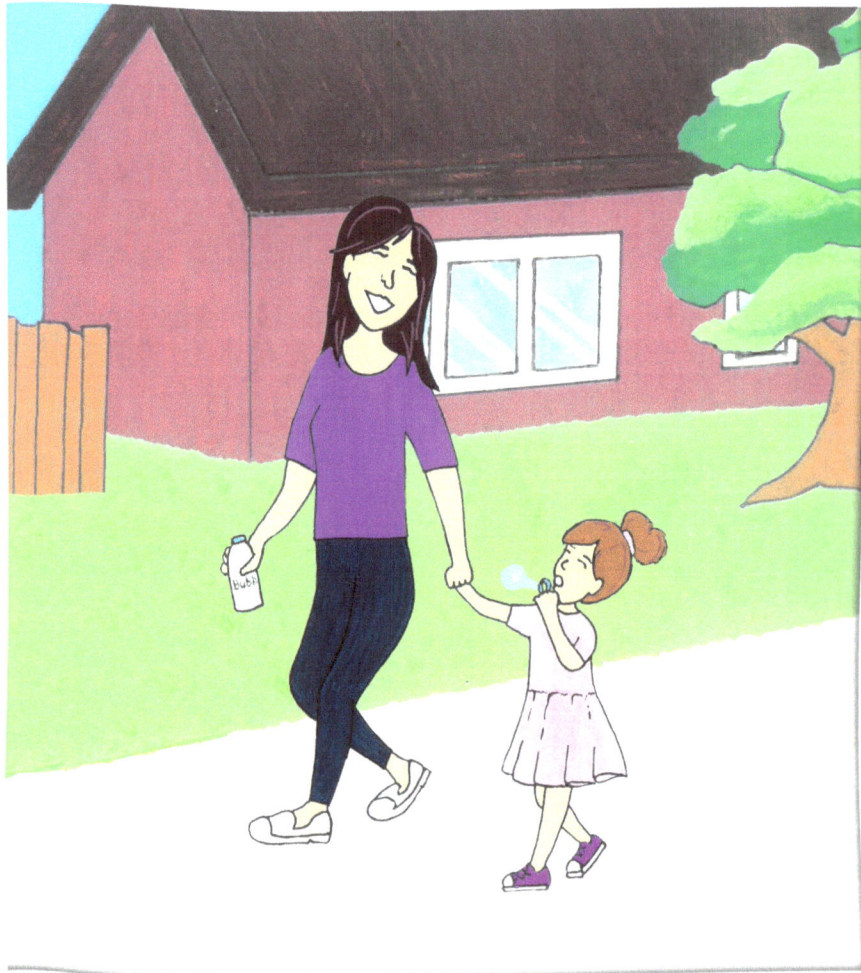